Your Pocket Therapist

Your Pocket Therapist

DR ANNIE ZIMMERMAN

First published in Great Britain in 2024 by Orion Spring,
an imprint of The Orion Publishing Group Ltd
Carmelite House, 50 Victoria Embankment
London EC4Y 0DZ

An Hachette UK Company

5 7 9 10 8 6 4

A CIP catalogue record for this book is available from the British Library.

All images from Shutterstock

ISBN (Hardback) 978 1 3987 1601 8
ISBN (Export Trade Paperback) 978 1 3987 1602 5
ISBN (eBook) 978 1 3987 1604 9
ISBN (Audio) 978 1 3987 1605 6

Printed and bound in India by Manipal Technologies Limited

Every effort has been made to ensure that the information in the book is accurate. The information in this book may not be applicable in each individual case so it is advised that professional medical advice is obtained for specific health matters and before changing any medication or dosage. Neither the publisher nor author accepts any legal responsibility for any personal injury or other damage or loss arising from the use of the information in this book. In addition if you are concerned about your diet or exercise regime and wish to change them, you should consult a health practitioner first.

www.orionbooks.co.uk

CONTENTS

PREFACE

All patient stories are fiction.

There is no perfect term for someone who comes to therapy – I find the word 'client' transactional and impersonal, so I prefer to use 'patient', as it implies a duty of care and a sense of being looked after, which feels important to me. For ease, then, I will use 'patient' throughout.

INTRODUCTION

I am sitting on a sofa in a warmly lit room, looking across to a wise face with inquisitive eyes. Everything is about to change. I fidget in the chair, as nervous as I would be before a first date – just not the kind of date you sneakily text your friends about when they've gone to the bathroom. No one knows I'm here actually. There's a sort of shame in telling people, as if they might think I'm crazy or broken for being here.

I'm not here because I've had a mental breakdown. Actually, I'm pretty sure my mental health is fine. If I'm honest, I'm not sure why I'm here. All I know is that I'm suffering and I don't know what else to try. I can't stop eating. No matter what diet I try, what new type of exercise I take up or food group I attempt to cut out, I'm stuffing my face until my belly hurts every single day. I eat in a frenzy until I feel sick, comatose on the sofa, barely present. I feel sluggish and ugly and miserable. Honestly, I don't think therapy is going to help at all. I'm just desperate.

I've tried everything. I've trawled through Google, downloaded a mindfulness app, started yoga, thought positively, wrote in a gratitude journal, worked harder to distract myself, talked exclusively about food, stopped talking about food completely. I've given up sugar, written notes of warning to myself, kept chocolate out of the house, skipped meals out with friends, counted to ten, counted to a hundred, had three meals a day, five meals, no meals. Sometimes things helped a little, but the problem always came back.

I have no idea why I'm struggling; I just know that I can't stop.

I look up at this woman who has listened to me ramble on about myself for an hour and ask, 'So, what on earth is wrong with me?'

'It sounds like you're in a lot of pain,' she says. 'Let's try to work it out together.'

We agree to meet once a week and I leave feeling unsure and sceptical that this will help, but for the first time in a long time, I have a tiny glimmer of hope that things might get better.

Fast-forward a few months and I find myself struggling to speak. My eyes are full. My body screams at me not to let her see me cry, but I breathe through the pain and let a tear fall. I look up to check she's not annoyed; she nods encouragingly. I am talking about something from my past that I've never told anyone before. I was seven and being shouted at for a reason I didn't quite understand. I went to the cupboard afterwards to make myself feel better. This was the first time I learnt to use food to comfort myself.

We talk, over many months, about everything other than food. It turns out that the reasons I started therapy have absolutely nothing to do with the things I end up talking about. I talk about my parents, about my sister, boyfriends, the mean girls at school. I talk about my desires, the things I'm afraid of, how I feel about myself. Yet somehow, without ever really talking about food, the problem shifts. It isn't just talking; I'm also crying, I'm angry, jealous, ashamed, humiliated, lonely and deeply, deeply sad. Before this I would have said I was fine – generally a happy person. Now I realise I am full of feeling.

Afterwards, I leave and the familiar urge to eat fills me. In the cupboard, I grab my go-to chocolate biscuits and then stop myself. 'Try to notice what's going on in your body,' I hear my therapist saying. There's a twinge of sadness. I stay with it for a moment and my eyes fill. I blink out a tear, then another.

My body takes me to bed and now I'm weeping. It feels good, like a cathartic release. After a few minutes, my tears dry and I feel vulnerable but a little better. I did not eat. The biscuits remain in the cupboard, untouched. A smile fills my face. There is nothing wrong with me. I am just very sad, and angry, and the eating has been keeping all that pain down. As I lie in bed, euphoria floods me. I thought it was the eating that was wrong with me, but I realise the eating was trying to make me feel better. The only thing that was wrong with me was that I didn't yet know what was going on emotionally for me underneath the surface.

That's when I realised that most of us don't have a clue why we are suffering. Most of our psychological problems are an attempt to cope with pain. The problems create a new kind of difficulty in our lives, but the initial root of the problem might be entirely unrelated.

This wasn't the end of the binge eating, but it was the start of the end. And, several years of hard work later, I can proudly say that it's a problem that rarely rears its ugly head. Now, when it does, I understand that it's a signal of a deeper issue. In those moments, I allow myself to look under the surface, with the same compassion my therapist showed me, and it goes away once more.

This groundbreaking realisation motivated me to become a psychotherapist. Every woman in my family is a therapist. Every single one. My mother is a therapist, my sister is a therapist, all four of my aunties are therapists. My grandma was one of the first women to study psychology at university in the UK. It's safe to say I've been raised in a cult of therapy.

So, it's no wonder I ended up completing a PhD in psychology and going on to train to become a psychotherapist. It's literally in my blood.

While this has at times been extremely irritating and makes family gatherings pretty heavy going, it's also given me a love and appreciation for the human condition, and a solid foundation of understanding about mental health and the way therapy works. Yet still, it was only in going through therapy and becoming a therapist myself that I came to understand that fundamental point: most of us have no idea what the real problem is.

In modern Western culture we tend to believe that our conscious mind is in the driving seat. In reality, however, it's our unconscious mind that runs the show. It determines how we react to things, why we're anxious, why we procrastinate, why we prefer men who treat us badly, why girls coming on too strong freaks us out, why we're driven at work, why we can't sleep, why we're a supportive friend, why we stuff ourselves with food even though we're full, why we think everyone hates us; why we think, feel and do anything.

Sigmund Freud described the mind as an iceberg – the conscious mind is the 10 per cent we see, but underneath there's another 90 per cent of the iceberg, which is our unconscious. And yes, Freud was a little problematic, sex-obsessed and used to take his patients on holiday (weird, right?), but some of his ideas were rather brilliant, and still hold up today.

So many of us walk around with these big issues we can't seem to solve because we have no idea where they're coming from. In my practice, I see many people who are struggling. They know things aren't going as well as they'd like, they know they're grappling with certain issues and they know they want things to change. What they don't understand is why, or what to do about it.

What I tell my patients, and what's essential for you to understand, is that you cannot change unless you get to the root of your problems. The things we *think* are the problems are often not the problems themselves. Food was a coping mechanism I'd learnt to make me feel better. It numbed me from deeper emotions that I wasn't even aware of. Food, in a counter-intuitive way, was a solution. For others, the solution might be different things – relationships, substances, work, self-criticism, anxiety, depression.

Your problems are signposts that something is going on underneath. They are the tip of the iceberg.

The tools people learn in therapy, and that you will learn in this book, help you take a look inside to see what's going on below the surface of the water. There's nothing that gives me more pleasure than seeing one of my patients have a moment of revelation, in which they realise something they've never made sense of before (or a therapiphany, as I like to call it). Sometimes these a-ha moments are a relief, often they are painful, but they are always necessary for deep transformation to occur.

Desperate to bring the life-changing insights that people learn in therapy outside of the therapy room, I sought to distil complex psychological concepts into simple and digestible posts on social media. Within a matter of months, my small group of followers became hundreds of thousands of people.

I couldn't believe how much my posts were resonating with people.

What this shows me is that people are hungry for depth and to really understand themselves. There is a growing movement, especially among young people, to engage on a more profound level with our mental health and a quiet revolution leading us away from oversimplification towards the pursuit of true self-awareness. People are yearning for answers.

This book will provide the depth we're craving by answering the questions people are longing to unpick by summarising the fundamentals of our psychology and relationships.

People come to therapy for all kinds of reasons, but the thing they all have in common is that they want something in their lives to change. There might be hundreds of different problems that people want to address, but fundamentally they feel stuck and want their life to improve.

Part of what keeps us stuck is that we're asking ourselves the wrong questions – questions that prevent us from moving forward. One of the first things they teach you in therapy school is that you don't have a magic pill or a simple answer that can just take away someone's problems. Trust me, if I had a magic wand, I would use it. What I can do is help people to ask different kinds of questions, which get underneath the tip of the iceberg. And they're the questions I'm going to ask you in this book.

It is not a substitute for therapy, but it is going to arm you with the tools to gain self-knowledge, so you can observe and learn about yourself. When you understand your reactions and behaviours, you give yourself a choice and power over your decisions.

This is the book I wish everyone would read before starting therapy or any healing journey. It's the book I wish I'd had before I started. Each chapter will answer the questions I get asked the most, by my patients and people online. It will be full of tips, stories, exercises and lessons in manageable, bite-sized pieces that will help to explain complex and otherwise inaccessible theory on relationships, how to become more self-aware, how to feel better and how to improve your life.

Because while therapy can be hugely transformative, we are really the masters of our own mind. And the more we empower ourselves with knowledge, the more successful our healing is likely to be.

There are five key steps in my process to understanding your emotions and moving past your suffering:

1. **GET CURIOUS:** recognise what the problem is, that it's signposting a deeper issue underneath, and start thinking about what that might be. When did the issue first develop? What role might it be serving? Think about how this shows up in your relationships and any patterns you've observed that keep cropping up.

2. **UNDERSTAND:** go deep into your past experiences, becoming more aware of what the root of the problem might be, and why it is there.

3. **FEEL:** experience the emotions that are being kept down. We are all very talented at avoiding things we don't want to face, even without realising.

4. **ACT:** turn this new awareness into action to make different choices.

5. **REPEAT:** notice when these patterns reoccur, go through these steps, then notice when it inevitably comes up again (and again and again and again).

This might sound simple, and really it is; however, it takes repetition and practise because our unconscious pain doesn't always want to be felt so readily. I don't want to delude you that this is a neat five-step process – therapy is anything but neat. Healing is not linear. You might bounce from getting curious to feeling, to going back into denial that there is a problem at all, to taking action, to feeling deeply again, to having a pause for a while and then going back to it when you feel stronger. There is no 'right' way to do this; the journey will look different for everyone, but these are the five fundamental aspects around which I find it useful to anchor the process. So don't be alarmed if the experience is messy. If you ever have the thought, *Am I doing this right?* please know that there is no right or wrong way – messiness just means you're human, like the rest of us.

I'm going to go through some of the main signposts that cause people suffering. We'll focus on both the self (e.g. depression, anxiety, obsessive thinking, addictions, self-criticism) and relationships (e.g. projection, why you can't get over your ex, how to stop pushing people away, loneliness, friendship break-ups, having difficult conversations). And along the way we're going to look at how to put all this self-knowledge into action, giving you practical tools so that you can start to understand why you are struggling, and how you can struggle less.

A NOTE BEFORE WE START

There's only one golden rule in my therapy room: my patients should say everything and anything that comes into their head. If they get a strange, embarrassing or seemingly random thought, I actively encourage them to say it. The same applies to you as you're reading this book. Any shameful, silly, out-of-nowhere thought, feeling or memory that comes up, I want you to allow it to be there, welcome it in and get curious. Maybe even write it down.

These random thoughts are often coming from the unconscious. They are communications from a part of yourself you're likely unaware of. By starting to pay attention to them, you're becoming more aware of these parts of yourself that have been hiding away, yet probably are having far more of an impact on your life than you realise.

Of course, if the things that come up feel too overwhelming, it's important to notice this, stay curious, but also maybe take a pause if you need to. If you do feel easily triggered, it might be a signal that there's something specific you're struggling to deal with that might require professional support.

When someone comes into my consulting room, I don't immediately know what's at the root of their suffering. They're telling me they often feel flat, that they've stopped having sex with their partner and they get these random headaches that they've convinced themselves is a brain tumour. This is where being a psychotherapist is a little like being a detective. I piece these bits of information together and begin to construct my own theories, based on things I've learnt, about why someone might have developed the coping mechanisms they're telling me about, but really, I don't know what's going on inside them. The journey of figuring it out is one we embark on together.

Just as my therapist didn't know exactly why I was binge eating at first – we had to uncover it together – I am likewise in the dark when a new patient arrives. So I start by asking questions about their life, their childhood, how they came to be.

Throughout this book I want you to play detective in your own life. Get curious. Where might certain beliefs have come from? What patterns do you observe? Is there something that seems to be repeated in different parts of your life?

You cannot heal if you aren't aware of what is broken

People often ask me, 'How do I heal?' and my answer is always, 'Self-awareness.' Awareness is the first step towards change. Until we know what we're dealing with, we don't know how to help ourselves. Once we are aware of the *what* and the *why*, we can take responsibility, challenge old patterns and start to make conscious changes. Without self-awareness, change is a struggle.

Remember that behaviours, patterns and habits serve a function, so you will have developed them for a reason or as a product of the unconscious things you've repressed, usually from your childhood. Beyond the signpost there is an opportunity for deeper understanding. Now you need to follow those signposts and try to understand exactly what's going on underneath.

I'm going to give broad examples of people struggling with each issue I describe in the book, what might be the source of them, and some tips and tools on what to do about it. This will be unique for everyone – while the problem might be similar, the root cause can be very different.

One person might struggle with social anxiety because their dad died when they were little, and their child mind wondered irrationally if it was something they had done – if he'd died because they were bad. Another person might have had a critical mother who left them scared of the judgement of others; another may have had to look after their younger siblings even though they were still a child and feel now that people are always wanting something from them.

I'm not here to tell you what the reasons are for your struggles; only you can know that. Instead, I'm going to provide you with the tools to start building more self-awareness around your problems and some routes for working through them. I'm here with you every step of the way. Let's start with an exercise to prepare you for the journey.

– *EXERCISE* –

I want you to play detective. As you read through each section, pay attention to how you feel. Are there any stirrings in your body? Any thumps of anxiety in your chest or twinges of sadness in your eyes? If this happens, put the book down and just notice the feeling. Give it space. See what happens. As you read, stay focused on how you feel – this is where the healing lies.

Any random thoughts, memories, feelings, odd sensations in your body – write them down. These are all unconscious communications that might give us more of a clue as to what's going on in there.

Give yourself a few minutes to reflect on anything you've already noticed. Do any more associations come up? Do these link to any of the issues you're having? Any new explanations or a-ha moments?

If you're getting nothing, that's fine too. Stay open-minded as we go through each section of the book and see where you might want to get curious and dig into what might be going on under the surface of your problems.

As you start playing detective, it's important for you to know that understanding yourself isn't about having an intellectual awareness of what's going wrong. You might well understand that the reason why you hate confrontation is because, for example, your mum used to be controlling and aggressive, which scared you. While this is an important insight, it won't change that fact. If it was that easy, you'd heal everything by reading one book on child development, and therapy would only last one session – you'd sit in the chair, the therapist would tell you it's all your mum's fault (which we definitely sometimes do), they'd explain that the difficulties you're having are ways you learnt to cope as a child and you'd leave problem-free, barely needing to make a dent in your bank account.

Unfortunately, it doesn't work like that, because what really needs to be understood are the feelings that have been kept out. Rather than just *knowing* that your mum's meanness made you scared of conflict, bit by bit you have to emotionally connect to what it really felt like for you at the time, how scary it was, what it was like to try to speak up. In order to make change, you have to release what's been repressed by going back to what it felt like to be that little child.

Understanding yourself is not so much about *knowing* why, but about *feeling* why.

I know this might seem scary. It was scary for me too. Delving into your past and letting yourself get sad or angry or afraid might be the last thing you want to do. It might feel genuinely terrifying. I can remember when I first started therapy, squirming away from the difficult parts, talking about things that were completely irrelevant or changing the subject when I could feel the stirring of a painful emotion or memory. If I'm honest, I still do that now sometimes, even though I know full well it won't help me. The unconscious will do anything to avoid being vulnerable if it feels that is threatening. This is completely normal.

There might be a moment when you read this and get irritated at something or think I'm talking nonsense. Be curious about that too. That happens often in therapy. When a comment hits a nerve, it's normally hitting something in your unconscious that you want to deny or avoid. If you can notice it rather than react to it, this could be a moment of insight that will help you to understand yourself better.

Take your time with this work. If you've gone all your life believing it's not safe to feel certain things and then a therapist comes along and asks you repeatedly how you're feeling, you're not suddenly going to say, 'No problem, I'll open up all my dark insides that I once thought were going to make my parents stop loving me, ultimately ending in death.' No. Even though you want to get better and probably very much want this person to know exactly how you're feeling, your unconscious is going to put up a good fight.

That's why the process of therapy can be a long one, because we gently have to teach the scared part of you that it is indeed safe to feel those things. And, much to the dismay of our quick-fix, magic-pill, instant-gratification culture, that takes as long as it takes.

So as you read, focus on what you're feeling. And remember, we're trying to *feel* our feelings, not *think* our feelings.

Part One:

THE SELF

Understanding Yourself

Most of us just want to be happy. Alva especially wants to be happy. She's spent her lifetime chasing happiness, yet somehow she cannot find it. She can't quite say why – nothing in her life is that bad – but she moves through her days like tar. She finds herself constantly scrolling through her phone, playing *Candy Crush* every moment she can. At family gatherings she zones out, her thoughts going round and round that she's failing in life, that nothing is working and everything is pointless. She feels happiness sometimes – dancing with friends, laughing at stupid videos, cuddling her cat – but the tar always returns.

She wakes up yet again with a heaviness in her limbs. Before she even opens her eyes, she feels for her phone to prepare herself for another day of dissatisfaction. Her thumbs open *Candy Crush*, an action as reflexive as breathing at this point. She looks at the clock. An hour has gone by; she's late for work and she's missed the workout class she promised herself she'd do in hopeful delusion the day before. With a frustrated groan, Alva throws her phone across the room. That's it, something has to change. Today is the day she is going to fix this problem – she's going to do everything she can to get happy.

She invests heavily in the happiness industry. She buys herself a new wardrobe, wondering if this will be the thing to make her happy. It doesn't. She deletes *Candy Crush* and sets limits on her apps. It works for a few days, but she always goes back to it. She starts a new health regime, trying to eat well and get into running. It gives her a smug sense of superiority, but it doesn't make her happy, not really. She quits her office job and goes travelling, spends a year in India, Mexico, Bali. She gets into yoga and feels a little better, but still the sorrow follows her.

Maybe she needs more meaning, more purpose. She changes career, retrains as a teacher, hoping that working with children will give her a sense of gratification. It does, but she still has this niggling feeling of deep sadness. Maybe what she needs is a relationship, someone to love and hold her. She meets Jamal. He's perfection – funny, sexy, ambitious and attentive. For a few months, it works. She's giddy and excited, everything feels a little brighter. When she's with him, she doesn't even think about her phone. Maybe this was the answer. Maybe her strange feeling of disconnection is finally gone.

Then, once the honeymoon period has calmed and the oxytocin (the 'love hormone') simmers down, the same nameless dread returns. She starts zoning out at work again. Going to meet her friends becomes laborious. She finds herself fake-laughing and saying she's fine a lot, but inside it's a different story. Her *Candy Crush* habit slips back in; she plays it on the bus, as soon as she wakes up, right before bed. She even starts playing when she's hanging out with Jamal, making them feel disconnected and alone. Once again, the world has lost its colour and Alva doesn't know why.

Why can't she just be happy? It's not like she isn't trying.

The problem is that Alva is not getting anywhere near the heart of the matter. All her attempts at problem-solving are hitting the tip of the iceberg. Now, don't get me wrong, your job, relationships and lifestyle have huge implications for your mental health, but they don't get deep into why you – and Alva – are struggling in the first place.

Desperate for things to change, Alva comes to see me. In our first session, I immediately sense how frightened she is to open up. The anxiety radiating from her is palpable. She is smiling but she does not seem happy. She seems distracted and aloof, tails off at the end of her sentences as if she's not used to talking about herself. She reminds me of myself when I first started therapy. Numb, scared and detached from herself. 'What do I do?' she asks. 'Tell me what to do.'

People come to therapy for answers, but often I start by giving them more questions (yes, therapists are annoying like that; you'll learn this as we go). I do not hold the answers. I wish I could give people the magic pill they're after – it would make my job a hell of a lot easier – but sadly no such thing exists. All the answers lie within Alva, but they're outside of her awareness at this point – the underside of the iceberg. My job is to help her feel safe enough to get to them.

So, together, we start the process of excavation.

The first thing I do is ask about her childhood – a cliché, I know.

Why are therapists obsessed with your childhood?

The majority of brain development happens between birth and three years, and the brain is nearly fully grown by the time we're five. This means that everything that happens to us during this time has deep consequences for who we become. Think about how we learn language: babies can pick up a new language easily and will stay largely fluent for the rest of their lives, whereas trying to learn a new language after the age of twelve is pretty hard for most of us.

As we learn how to speak, we also learn a language of emotions. Most of what we know about ourselves, our relationships and the world comes from those early years.

Sadly, we are evolved for survival, not for happiness. Your brain does not care that your social media addiction is turning you into a zombie, or that your inability to motivate yourself is stopping you from doing well at work. Your brain just wants to protect you from things it deems to be potentially harmful.

And where do we learn what's harmful to our survival? Our childhood.

As an adult you might be able to feed and look after yourself, but as a child this was certainly not the case. This is truer for us in comparison to any other species because we are so helpless as babies. We spend the first two years of our lives completely dependent on others to survive, needing them to feed us, hold us and stop us from rolling off tables.

For a baby to stay alive, it needs to maintain the connection to its parents. It needs to be loved.

So as babies we are hyper-attuned to things that strengthen or weaken our relationships. When a parent is not present, shouts at us or is highly stressed, this sends out fear signals in our brain. This feeling of fear tells us something is wrong, and as babies we try everything we can to fix it and keep our parents happy. We need them to keep us alive, and for that we need them to love us. Anything that we perceive will make them love us more gets ramped up, and anything we think will make them stop loving us gets shoved down.

Even if your parents were emotionally literate and non-judgemental, you would have implicitly learnt what's socially acceptable by osmosis from your environment. Men shouldn't cry; women shouldn't be assertive; we should be confident but not proud, happy but not arrogant. It's in our cultural make-up – and will vary depending on which culture, race, class and country we're from. There is an endless list of messages we get from society about who we *should* be, how we *should* act, what we *should* think. Take the messages we receive about our feelings alone: 'Think positively', 'Don't be glum', 'Man up', 'Just get on with it', 'Put on a brave face', 'Don't be a wimp', 'Big boys don't cry', 'Keep calm and carry on'. So, it's not just your immediate family that shapes you; it's also wider society, your culture, sexuality, race, class, religion, neurotypicality – the list goes on. As we grow, all of these experiences of living in the world shape how we learn to relate to people, and ourselves.

Any feelings, behaviours or identities that have elicited negative responses get pushed down into the unconscious, where we have no real awareness that we even have them.

That's why bad things that happen to you when you are young have such a significant effect on you as an adult. Adverse childhood experiences (ACEs) are the leading predictor of poor mental and physical health, from anxiety to heart disease. The more difficult our childhoods were, the worse we will suffer.

ACEs

'The Adverse Childhood Experiences (ACE) Study'[1] found that patients who experienced four or more types of adverse childhood events had higher rates of ischaemic heart disease, cancer, stroke, chronic bronchitis, emphysema, diabetes and hepatitis. Extensive research has shown that ACEs also increase the risk of mental health conditions, with one in three of them relating to ACEs. Results are so stark that childhood maltreatment is shown to be the costliest health issue in the United States, while resolving child abuse would improve the rate of depression by over half, alcoholism by two-thirds, and suicide, serious drug abuse and domestic violence by three-quarters.[2]

But my childhood was great!

It may well have been, but it still had an impact on you. Now, let me be clear. We have all been let down by our parents in big and small ways, and this has, to varying degrees, messed us up. Even those with the most emotionally attuned, caring and well-adjusted parents will have experienced some negative moments that probably still affect them today.

Below are some experiences that aren't considered trauma but still affect a child:

- The birth of a younger sibling and losing your parents' sole attention.
- Mum working a lot.
- Dad not talking much about his feelings.
- Being picked on in class.
- Going to boarding school and being separated from your family.
- Getting the silent treatment.
- Being encouraged to be happy all the time rather than being allowed to be sad.
- High expectations or pressure to achieve in school.
- Living in a dangerous area with violence around you.
- Growing up in a culture that's different from the people around you.
- Moving around a lot.

If you recognise any of these things from your childhood, it might feel weird or scary to think of yourself as having been negatively impacted by your upbringing. Maybe you want to dismiss me and tell me how lovely your parents were (I don't doubt it). It's difficult to think about our childhoods being anything other than good, but good is not the full spectrum of feelings. Things can be good and still hard at times. We can love people and still be upset with them. The more shades we can admit and accept, the more we can understand ourselves and feel whole.

There are two types of trauma: small-t trauma and big-T trauma. Big-T traumas are normally life-threatening or intensely frightening – such as physical or sexual abuse. Small-t traumas aren't quite as terrible, but they can still be distressing. These are experiences that we might not classify as big-T trauma, but they can threaten a child's sense of safety and therefore be experienced as traumatic.

Trauma is defined as anything that shatters our sense of security in both our internal and external worlds. It is the emotional and physical response that comes from experiencing a distressing event. In other words, when bad things happen, our trust in our sense of safety is broken. In Greek, the word trauma means wound – so trauma isn't the event itself, it is how we process that event and how we store it within our psyche. This means that children can have the exact same experience, but (depending on their sensitivity, genes, family support, culture) one can be traumatised by it and one can be relatively OK.

The healing journey for those who have suffered severe abuse and trauma will no doubt be more complicated and painful than for those who haven't, but this is a spectrum, and everyone falls onto it somewhere. No matter how good or bad things have been for you, your childhood shaped you in positive and negative ways, and is still affecting you today as an adult. Self-awareness and understanding around exactly how is beneficial.

It's hard to think and talk about our childhoods. I get it – it took me about a year of therapy to admit that my parents were anything other than flawless (and I still sometimes find myself getting defensive about it). We can feel guilty for being critical; our parents did so much for us – we shouldn't complain or blame them. Contrary to what you might have heard about therapists, I'm not here to blame your parents.

They did the best they could. However, being defensive about whether they were or were not good parents shuts down any curiosity about who you are and what you could learn about yourself and the world.

Let's leave the blame here, and instead get curious.

– EXERCISE–

Imagine yourself as a child – any age that comes to mind. What kind of child were you? Are you aware of anything that might have been difficult for you? This can be something as seemingly inoffensive as a family dog dying or going to a new school. Put yourself in the mind of a child – what might that have felt like for you back then?

What about your relationships? Were there any that were difficult? Even if you were a really happy kid with loving parents, were there any less-than-ideal dynamics to your relationships with your family? We can't all be happy all the time; it's natural to have a whole range of more difficult feelings. How might that have been for that little kid?

If you're struggling to find answers, try to think of your earliest memory. What was going on in your family at the time? What might it tell you about the kind of childhood you had?

Asking yourself these questions allows us to start piecing together what might be buried in your unconscious. Without blame or judgement towards your parents, we can start to try to figure out the experiences and attachments that shaped who you are.

Back to Alva . . .

I don't get anywhere with Alva very fast. She zones out often and I feel a bit like I don't really exist when I'm with her, as if she's in a glass box that she's keeping me out of. I try to connect with her, to empathise and understand what she's feeling, but she is mostly numb, and therefore so am I. My attempts to connect only seem to push her further inwards.

So, I start to ask Alva the same questions I've just asked you in an attempt to figure out where she learnt to disconnect, and what exactly she's disconnecting from. As she tells me about her childhood – in a monotonous, detached tone – I start to get more of a picture of where her disconnect might have come from. She tells me that her dad used to get in bad moods. I ask her to give me an example, to see if she can remember what this used to feel like and also to connect her to the feelings it seems as though she's shutting me – and herself – out from.

A six-year-old Alva is playing with a football in the garden outside, kicking it against the wall back and forth. *Thwack. Thwack.* Dad is at the kitchen table trying to focus on his work. *Thwack.* He glances out of the window and tries to re-read the sentence. *Thwack.* His jaw tenses. *Thwack.* That's it. Dad loses it. He storms into the garden. 'Shut up! Stop that right now. Why do you have to be so damn annoying?' Alva freezes in fear at the shock. Her jaw clenches. She was only playing; she didn't do anything wrong. She turns to her dad to shout back, but he is big and red and frowny. Her lips tremble. It's the first time she has seen her dad like this; normally he's loving and smiley. Panic rises through her. What if he shouts more? What if he thinks she's bad and stops loving her? Scared and wanting the shouting to stop, she apologises, stops playing with the ball and goes inside to play a game on the computer.

This doesn't mean Alva didn't feel angry and hurt at being told off when she was innocently playing, it just didn't feel safe for her to show her feelings at the time in case it made her dad more mad and ultimately stop loving her, which you'll remember is a child's greatest fear. Instead, the anger and hurt got pushed down. And turned against herself.

This kind of thing started to happen often when Alva was a child. After a few occasions, she got so used to pushing her anger down that she stopped being aware of it bubbling up. That doesn't mean the anger had gone; it was just repressed in the unconscious.

When she went inside to play video games, she realised that it made her feel a little better. She was still upset and angry, but the game released pleasure hormones, which made her feel temporarily better. The next time Alva's dad shouted, and she was too scared to shout back, she went to play computer games again to suppress her big feelings.

By the time she became an adult her anger and fear were completely repressed. In fact, she tells me she's the kind of person who doesn't get angry. But she also tells me she spends hours playing video games, scrolling on her phone, and watching porn and masturbating. She finds herself almost constantly numb and disconnected, with no real understanding of why.

As she tells me all this, a warmth fills my chest. It's the first time I've really felt loving towards her. This feels important, that she's letting me in, letting me see her vulnerability. I lean in, and she looks up at me, scared and small. Of course Alva still needs to use video games to soothe herself and keep her difficult feelings down. Inside is a little girl who is afraid and angry but isn't allowed to be.

Our parents teach us how to feel

Children are incredibly sensitive to how their parents deal with emotions. There might not have been any direct communication that you shouldn't feel certain feelings, but you might have picked up on the fact that some were more acceptable than others.

You might have learnt to repress your feelings because:

- your parents didn't show their feelings or talk about emotions much.
- your parents were always encouraging you to be happy and think positively.
- your mum was very anxious and easily upset; you felt she was too fragile to upset further.
- your father was very sensitive to criticism, so he interpreted your tantrums as personal attacks that made him give you the silent treatment.
- you had a loud and dominating younger sibling, and your parents didn't have space for two problem children, so you learnt that being smiley and quiet got you more love and attention.
- bad things happened but were never talked about; everything was pushed under the carpet.
- you had to look after your younger siblings, even though you were still a child yourself.
- you were bullied in school, taught to 'man up' and be strong otherwise you'd be seen as weak.

In these situations, over time we learn that our natural feelings of sadness, anger, envy and hatred will stop us from receiving love. While it's very normal to feel annoyed or upset with our parents, it might not feel safe to show these feelings because we need their love and attention to survive.

This is where things start to go wrong for our mental health. The beliefs stored in our unconscious mind were created when we were children and first learning about the world. We developed them based on the things that kept us safe when we were young. We might have learnt that when we cry, adults get angry and tell us to stop, so crying became risky. Maybe we were laughed at when we did a presentation in school, so we learnt that public speaking isn't safe because it makes us feel excluded and humiliated. Maybe our parents weren't very good at talking about feelings, so they shut down when we tried to say how we felt, which was scary. You might not be consciously aware of any of this; you might find you just feel very uncomfortable when you have to give a talk at work, or when someone forces you into a conversation about feelings.

All these lessons about what's safe and what's not create limiting beliefs that are stored in our unconscious and provide a compass for our adult lives without us realising. We might believe we aren't good enough, so we sabotage our new job opportunity. Maybe we don't believe we're worthy of love, so we push away people who treat us well in favour of those who treat us badly. Maybe we believe it isn't safe for other people to be angry at us, so we live our lives doing everything we can not to upset people.

The Internal Saboteur

Self-sabotage often comes from the inner critic we all have – which is normally formed from the negative judgements of others and society. The psychoanalyst Ronald Fairbairn called this our 'internal saboteur'[3]. The saboteur is trying to protect us from being shamed or rejected by others. It might have started off as a protector that we needed to survive threatening situations when we were younger, but as an adult, the saboteur tends to do more harm than good because the threats are no longer there. The saboteur part keeps reminding us of the things we've done wrong, catastrophises about the future, avoids certain situations, ruins relationships and opportunities. It's not actively trying to make our life miserable; it's trying to keep us from being hurt in the ways we've been hurt before, but the very thing that once kept us safe is now the cause of our suffering and inertia.

Self-sabotage is a signpost that there's something going on in your unconscious that's calling the shots. Rather than blaming yourself, try to get curious about what's going on.

Other examples of self-sabotage:

What's happening: **you really want to start a new exercise regime, but never make it to the gym.**
What might be happening underneath: **deep down you might not believe you deserve to take care of yourself. Or you don't like feeling uncomfortable, or you're afraid to be bad at something, so you don't try.**

What's happening: **you say you want to be more open but swerve every emotional conversation.**
What might be happening underneath: **maybe you're very afraid of being vulnerable.**

What's happening: **you say you're unhappy in your job but find reasons why you can't leave or mess up your job opportunities.**
What might be happening underneath: **happiness or having the thing you want feels scary because it might get taken away. There is safety in staying with something familiar even if it's making you miserable, and danger in leaving and trying something new and unknown.**

Rather than thinking of this behaviour as something that's ruining things for us, maybe we can think of it as something that is trying to help us. It's just got a warped understanding of what help is.

– *EXERCISE* –

Think of feelings you don't tend to feel – maybe you never get angry or haven't cried in years. What was the culture around that feeling in your family? Did your caregivers ever show their feelings?

Now think of any feelings you're not familiar with at all. Were they shown in your family? What response might you have got if you showed that feeling? Were there any consequences, i.e. would someone get upset or encourage you to feel more positively?

What's wrong with keeping things in?

If we avoid talking or thinking about the things that have happened to us, it keeps us mentally stuck. A friend described this to me as taking a bunch of dirty, wet clothes and shoving them in a cupboard because you don't want to deal with them. In a way they're dealt with because they're out of sight, but they're festering in there, growing mouldy and stinky as they sit there, the smell permeating your surroundings just as your unprocessed feelings permeate your life. You might not want to take them out and wash them – it might be painful and difficult to deal with them – but ultimately you need to deal with the mess to stop it from getting worse.

For the people reading this thinking, 'I feel EVERYTHING; if anything, I have too many feelings – I'm not pushing anything down,' it may sound strange but even you are probably keeping things down without realising. It's not just feelings in the unconscious, but also thoughts and memories. Too much feeling is usually about not being able to soothe yourself and needing other people to regulate your feelings for you. I'll cover this more in Chapter 2: Anxiety (see page 63), but please know that just because you're feeling a lot, it doesn't mean you aren't also avoiding things (not necessarily intentionally, of course).

Things that happen when you avoid things:

- You have lots of physical health issues, such as constant flus and colds.
- You struggle to relax.
- You feel numb, tired and depressed.
- You see yourself as a pretty chilled person, but then find yourself overreacting or blowing up at small things.
- You have low self-esteem.
- You have many racing thoughts, often feeling very anxious but unable to stop worrying.
- You're constantly distracted – by TV, drinking, over-eating, working. You don't like being alone with your thoughts.
- You don't often cry or get angry.
- You suffer with addiction.
- You create rituals to avoid feelings.
- You tend to self-sabotage or engage with self-destructive behaviours.
- You feel lonely even when with people, as if no one really knows you.
- You can't be in the moment and often have brain fog and feel absent-minded.

It's important to know that most of the time we are not aware that we're pushing feelings down. It all happens outside of our control. Alva has no idea that she's terrified and angry; she just gets the urge to stare at her phone or play *Candy Crush*.

I see many people who suffer with no awareness that they're repressing anything. I also see people who aren't even aware of the extent to which they are suffering.

Some of you may be reading this and thinking, 'But there's nothing really wrong. My life is lovely, my childhood was great; I just have some low-level anxiety, am overworked and underpaid, have a mild addiction to social media and wine, keep getting ghosted and there's this voice in my head that keeps telling me what a mess I am. Apart from that, I'm all good.'

A friend once told me he has '100 per cent mental health'. At the time, he was also a borderline alcoholic with severe insomnia who was unable to maintain a romantic relationship. What was interesting to me was that he didn't connect any of these things to his mental health or even his psychology. Many people think that mental health refers to specific disorders such as schizophrenia or bipolar disorder; however, we all have our mental health to look after, and a lot of the symptoms that let us know something isn't quite right can be far more subtle.

Here is a list of things I would categorise as being related to the mind:

- Biting your fingernails.
- Poor sleep.
- Obsessing about a person you've only been on one date with.
- Gut problems.
- Work stress.

- Cheating on partners.
- Chronic fatigue.
- Shouting at your children and then feeling guilty.
- Overthinking.
- Random headaches.
- Overeating.
- Impotence.

You might recognise some of these things in yourself as you're reading this. Don't be alarmed – this doesn't mean you're broken; it just means you're human. We all have our own mental health in the same way that we all have our own physical health.

As we go through the common problems we all face in the following pages, I will ask you to suspend any scepticism and, instead of insisting you're fine, try to think about some of the experiences and emotions that might be coming up for you from below the surface.

Tips to understand what's going on under the surface

1. **Get curious.** Reflect on any thoughts, images or memories that come into your mind, even if they seem completely unrelated or weird. These kinds of thoughts are often coming from the unconscious. By noticing any themes or patterns that come up, you can spot clues as to what might be going on inside. Try not to judge yourself or dismiss thoughts that feel irrelevant – often these are the very ones with the most meaning. I encourage you to write them down as you go.

2. **Understand.** Think back to your past. Try to remember what it was like for you as a child, and any particularly difficult memories that come up. To understand the root of our suffering, we have to go backwards to where it started. How were you taught to handle your feelings? What role did you take on in your family? Where did you learn to behave in the way you do? Keep remembering as you read. The past, and how it shows up in the present, is the key to self-awareness.

3. **Feel.** Pay attention to your body. Our minds might not be aware of the things we're keeping down, but our bodies often are. Feelings are physical sensations, so try to notice anything going on in your body as you read and give space to anything that comes up. Sometimes, if you're feeling stressed or uncomfortable, stopping to work out why and simply naming the feeling can help you feel a little better, even without doing anything about it.

DEPRESSION

Why Do I Feel Down?

Everyone knows George as a happy person. He's one of those people you think have it all sorted: crisp shirts, shiny shoes and charmingly floppy hair. On the whole, he does have it all sorted, or so he thinks. He's always up for a laugh with his mates, is a loving partner to his new wife and has a respectable job where he's considered a well-liked member of the team.

One day, soon after the wedding, his wife announces over breakfast that she's pregnant. They do a happy dance in the kitchen; everything is going exactly how he planned. Then, over the next few months, George finds he doesn't feel as excited as he thought he would. In fact, he doesn't feel much at all. He wakes up tired, with a kind of fog behind his eyes. He often struggles to get to sleep, but it's the kind of bone-deep fatigue that no amount of sleep can resolve. His boss puts him on a new, more high-profile project, and he doesn't get his usual buzz. This would have been the kind of thing that excited him before, but he finds now that he doesn't really care. He stops putting the extra work in, cancels on his friends at the pub, wants to do nothing other than sit in front of the television. Getting up for work becomes arduous, he stops wanting to have sex, food doesn't give him the same pleasure, even getting up to shower feels effortful.

He tells no one, too ashamed that they'll judge him for being anything other than happy about the baby. He takes his solace in the shower – the only place where he can break down without shame because the water disguises the tears that stream down his face every morning. When he is alone and in private, he wonders, 'What the hell is wrong with me?'

What's going on with George?

Feeling down is a normal part of being human, yet feeling down all the time (when there are more bad days than good) drains the colour from your life, as it did for George. When depression hits it can seem completely random and unwarranted. I see many people who question why they feel depressed when they know they have a lot of privilege or everything in their life is going OK. This is because the real reason for depression is hidden from us – it is buried in the unconscious, currently too unbearable to be felt. The problem is that often, when some negative feelings are pushed down, other positive feelings get pushed down too, so we're left with an absence of feeling. Our mind numbs us so we don't feel the negative emotion, but it numbs us to everything else too, so we don't feel much joy or pleasure either.

What does 'feel your feelings' actually mean?

You might have heard therapists – and most of the internet – telling you to *feel your feelings*, but what does this even mean? What do you do with feelings if not feel them?

Feelings are energy in the body. (Anyone remember the golden rule of physics from school? Energy cannot be created or destroyed, only transferred from one form or place to another.) E-motion = energy in motion. An emotion or a feeling is simply the experience of energy moving through the body. For example, when we feel excited we might get butterflies in our stomach; when we feel afraid our throat might constrict and our heart might beat faster; sadness feels like heaviness and tears; anger makes us hot and red and alert. Ever have a big cry and feel exhausted afterwards? That's because of all the energy that's been expended in having the feeling.

So what happens when we try to keep our feelings in? Even MORE energy is needed to squash them all down. Think about all those feelings as energy that is trying to come up, thrashing, squirming, jumping, exploding, wanting desperately to be set free. To keep this energy in requires a lot of effort, as if you're continuously pushing down on a box filled with forces that are pushing upwards. You're going to be pretty damn tired after that. Repressing our feelings uses up an enormous amount of energy, which can cause depression due to the energy lost in pushing them all down for so many years.

Depression isn't only about numbness, though; it's also about physical exhaustion and low motivation. A good metaphor for this is imagining pushing on both the brakes and the accelerator of a car at the same time. The car might not go anywhere, but you're still going to use a lot of petrol. Without even realising it, we do the exact same thing when we bottle our emotions, which leaves us exhausted, numb and low in mood.

This is where therapy or a good healing practice helps us to bear what feels unbearable so we can stop numbing ourselves and allow the feeling in. When we can start to process these feelings, the energy used up to repress them is released and the depression can start to lift.

How do you feel your feelings?

Some feelings we know we're pushing away, like when we feel a sensation of discomfort, so we go for the glass of wine, knowing it'll quiet that upsetting thought. Other feelings are so buried away that we don't register we're having them at all.

There are many ways to connect to your deeper feelings. Here are three practical things you can do:

- **Connect to your body.** To get to both the more surface-level and the deeper feelings, we have to listen to our body. Feelings are just physical sensations, remember? To tune in to your feeling is to tune in to your body. In the therapy room I ask my patients often what they're feeling in their body – whether there's any sensation of discomfort. Some people feel nothing, others feel their legs shaking, a knot of tension in their chest or a thumping in their head. I then ask them to give the feeling a shape or colour. Are there any associations that come up? Does it have an image that goes with it? A word? Does it *link to a memory? When was the earliest time in their life they had this feeling? You can do this for yourself – it's known as 'free* association'. How does your body feel right now? If you struggle to connect, give yourself a second to check in with yourself. Your body will tell you how it feels; you just need to give it the space.

Free Association

Free association is a common psychoanalytic technique that can be used to get in touch with the unconscious by allowing a person to express thoughts, feelings and memories without censoring or judging. When you allow the mind to wander without filtering, by verbalising whatever comes into your mind, without consciously analysing, we give space for unconscious memories or emotions to come up. Associating and visualising feelings in this way can be helpful in connecting to them on a more physical level, exploring any early memories of those feelings that can help us understand why we might struggle with them.

- **Journaling.** Another way to connect to your feelings is by journaling. When you sit down with a pen and paper, it's important to let yourself write freely without censoring what you say. This will allow your true thoughts to come out. Writing without planning or screening what we say can allow our unconscious feelings to be exposed through our words. You might be surprised by what you read back.

- **Breathwork.** Breathwork refers to breathing exercises and specific breathing techniques, such as holotropic breathwork, which usually recommends a pattern of breathing fast that can help with emotional release. Holotropic breathwork was developed in the 1970s by Stanislav Grof, an expert in transpersonal psychology and consciousness research. It increases oxygen in the body, which can move stuck emotions and help to release stress, bringing the body back to a calm state. Stanislav's wife, Christina Grof, ran workshops where people would engage in the breathwork and have powerful emotional release – sobbing, screaming, banging on the floor. It might sound mad, but actually the Grofs found that breathwork helps people to get out of their conscious mind, so suppressed thoughts and emotions can move towards the surface and be released. A meta-analysis of studies in 2023 supported Grof's observations, showing that breathwork can significantly improve stress and mental health.[4] If you're trying breathwork for the first time, I would recommend seeking out a class or a coach who can introduce you to some of these exercises to ensure you feel safe throughout if any uncomfortable emotions arise.

Often people find when beginning this process of feeling their feelings properly that things seem to get a little worse before they get better. That's because to really heal you have to go through all the painful emotions you have been avoiding. It's like taking those dirty clothes out of the cupboard and finally dealing with them. It might not be pleasant while you're doing it, but it's better than leaving them to grow mouldy in the cupboard.

You have to come to terms with parts of yourself you might not have wanted to accept. Being vulnerable is scary, especially if you've been taught it isn't safe. Be gentle with yourself and let whatever you're feeling come up. It's scary, but feelings don't last forever; they will move through you – you just have to let them.

Reach Out

If you are struggling with depression and suicidal thoughts, talking and expressing the pain you're in can be really helpful. That's why it's so important to reach out to someone – a friend, therapist or your GP. If you're in crisis and need to talk right now, you can contact 24-hour helplines with people who are ready to listen and can help you make sense of how you're feeling. The contact numbers for the Samaritans, National Suicide Prevention Helpline UK, and the text service Shout (if you'd prefer not to talk on the phone) are listed at the back of this book.

How does George get better?

For the first time in George's life, thoughts of ending his life start to occupy him. It scares him; he's always thought of himself as a happy person who loves life; he never thought he'd be the kind of person to contemplate suicide. He knows then that something isn't right and plucks up the courage to admit what's been going on to his wife. Later that night, they search for a therapist together, both relieved and a little frightened of what's to come.

The first few sessions feel strange to George and he doesn't think it is helping. He tells his wife it's a waste of their time and money. I can feel his frustration that I don't have answers for him – he wants me to wave a magic wand that makes him feel better, but I keep going back to his childhood, which he says was lovely. The scenes he describes are idyllic – his family is close, his parents are still together, there was lots of play and laughter and love. He assures me that is not the source of the problem.

Maybe he's right; maybe I've found someone whose upbringing really was perfect. Then in one session, as he's confessing about crying in the shower, his younger sister calls. 'Do you mind if I get that?' he says. 'It's probably urgent if it's her.' I nod, interested to see where this goes. He answers the phone like a worried parent, asking repeatedly if she's OK, if she needs help. I'm confused because from everything he's told me about his sister, she's a capable and independent person, a lawyer in the city with a family of her own. I wonder if something's wrong.

'Is everything OK?' I say to him as he finishes the call. 'You sound very concerned for her.'

'Oh, yeah, she's fine. We're just really close.' There's tension in his voice. I'm not sure exactly why, but I get the sense that there are more complicated feelings involved here beyond the lovely close relationship he describes.

'On the phone you sounded as if you were her parent, like you were looking after her.'

George sighs deeply, as people often do before they tell you about the Big Thing – the moment that changed the way they looked at the world forever.

His sister was born with complications and needed lots of care in her first year of life. He was only four and already feeling upset about having to share his mum and dad's attention; now he had to watch them frantic with anxiety about their premature daughter. 'That must have been so hard for you,' I say, trying to get to the pain I can sense underneath. George does not want my empathy. He insists that his sister was the one with the problems. I ask him to tell me more about what it was like for him, and he snaps – it was fine, it's got nothing to do with anything any more – a strong, defensive door-slam in my face. Where there is defensiveness there is usually pain lurking underneath. I drop it for now, making a note to come back to his sister when he's ready.

If you don't feel your feelings, someone else feels them for you

Feelings that are unexpressed get picked up on by others. As a therapist, the most important thing to do is to check in continuously with how you feel around the person you're talking to. When George was in my room, I often felt very sad. The sadness came out of nowhere; I'd be in a perfectly pleasant mood before he arrived. Then, minutes into the session, I'd find myself with tears in my eyes, having to suck my cheeks to stop from crying. George would be feeling nothing.

This is how I start to piece together what it is that George might be avoiding. When he talked about his sister I was aware of my reaction, that I felt deeply sad for him. It isn't the same for everyone. Around some people I might feel angry, flat, inferior, jealous, afraid, or sometimes disconnected and numb. If they aren't feeling but I am, it's usually a clue that the feelings they evoke in me are the ones they're not feeling in themselves.

Getting to the root

Eventually George reveals more about his sister's illness. Everything changed after she got sick. His parents were preoccupied with her, so much so that it seemed (to his child self) that they stopped caring about him. They started staying at the hospital for long stints while he was left with a nanny. They didn't laugh at his jokes any more or play with him like they used to. George was told to be a big boy, to be brave for his little sister, so that's what he did. He made it his mission to cheer his parents up and kept any feelings of jealousy, sadness or fear to himself.

His sister got better and things rebalanced; that difficult year was hardly mentioned again, forgotten in the fabric of their family story.

As we talk this through, we come to realise that his wife's pregnancy might have triggered unconscious memories of the birth of his sister, and the loss of love he felt from his parents. At first, he feels very guilty and resists my annoying insistence that he feels anything but joy about the impending birth of his child. But after a while he admits that inside there's a stirring – his chest is tight and his fingers feel fizzy when he talks about his sister. He feels bad for feeling jealous of his sister because she was sick; it wasn't her fault. I remind him he was a child, that his feelings were understandable, that it must have been a hard time for him. His eyes fill. For the first time, he lets himself cry. As we try to connect his past to his present he realises that, unconsciously, he's been worried that his wife will stop caring about him when the baby is born, just as it felt like his mum did. He's never told anyone this before, and his hands are shaking as he says it – his whole body screaming at him not to – but when he was little he sometimes used to wish she'd never been born. He used to imagine big books slamming on top of her or the dog eating her.

'Does that make me a terrible person?' he asks. 'Is there something terribly wrong with me?'

There is, of course, nothing wrong with George. George is processing all the unbearable feelings that weren't felt at the time. The feelings have been pushed under the surface, where they've lain dormant for most of his life. The pregnancy triggered all the unconscious memories and feelings of his sister's birth, which (emotions = energy, remember) required a huge amount of power to push down. This is why George felt down and heavy and lacking in motivation. The repression of all those feelings was completely exhausting him.

When George first walked through the door, I didn't have the answers. I could never have known that this was the cause of his depression, because George himself didn't know it. Together we were detectives, following the feeling to the source of the original wound.

*

In time, as the feelings and memories start to come up, George starts to feel a little better, a little lighter. It's not just *feeling* the feelings that help him, but *feeling* them with someone else there, showing him it's safe to be vulnerable, that he can express himself without it burdening others as he feared when he was young and sensed his parents didn't have space for him to be the one who wasn't OK. Therapy gives George the space to be the one in need, a space where he doesn't have to be good or strong, where he can safely have these feelings and learn that nothing terrible happens when he does.

We don't see each other for a few weeks when his daughter is born. Over the break I'm a little worried for him – how's he going to feel once she's born? Is his depression going to get worse or is he going to find a way to allow and express his complicated feelings so he can connect to his new child?

I breathe a sigh of relief when I see the smile on his face as he walks through the door. George is OK. Then I realise maybe I'm needing him to be happy, just like all the other people in his life, so I try to stay neutral and give space for what George is feeling – good or bad.

'Well . . .' he says.

'Well,' I reply.

'I'm completely in love.'

A rush of relief fills the room. George beams, and I can tell he means it. I can feel it from the way he keeps talking about her, showing me pictures and fawning over little things, like how she giggles in her sleep. He also feels terrified. As his capacity for feeling grows, he's connected to both immense love and immense fear. During our break he started to talk to some of his friends about it, and even his wife. Sometimes, when she's preoccupied with their daughter and forgets to ask how his big meeting at work went, he feels rejected and bitter, and the depressed feeling returns. Remembering the dirty washing in the cupboard, he tries to admit to himself, and to me, how he's really feeling – that he's jealous of his baby getting his wife's undivided attention, an irrational sense of unfairness at the loss of the attention. He knows these feelings come from a hurt, child place, and he knows there's nothing wrong with him for feeling that way. He tells her, without blaming or criticising her, that he's feeling rejected and together they deal with it. George is able to take ownership of his feelings, so they don't take ownership of him.

This is what happens on a good day; on a bad one, when neither of them has had much sleep, George reverts to old coping strategies, goes into a sulk, and the low feeling returns. After all, he's only human and is a work in progress, as we all are.

– *EXERCISE* –

It's time for you to play detective again. I want you to think of a period in your life where you've felt a little like George. Not necessarily depressed, but struggling with motivation, feeling low and generally not feeling like yourself. What was happening during this time in your life? Were there any events (even happy ones), changes, significant moments? What do you think could have been triggered in your unconscious?

Remember, there are no wrong or right answers – we're just being curious. Rather than punishing yourself for feeling low, telling yourself you should be working harder or feeling happier all the time like everyone on Instagram seems to be, just bring gentle curiosity to what might be going on underneath.

What if I can't find a reason for feeling low?

Depression can really just be an absence of feeling. I don't want to mislead you with George's story – there isn't always a clear 'a-ha' moment or neat explanation for why one might be depressed. There may not be a clear reason from your past that's obvious; it might be more of a general emotional shut down.

When things get overwhelming the nervous system can go into freeze mode. Chronic stress and difficult events that happen can feel like danger, which triggers us to shut down. It's like the fuse gets overwhelmed and our body short-circuits.

Freezing is a response to threat, similar to flight or fight, which can look like depression. The body and mind shut down (playing dead), stopping us from communicating, taking action or feeling.

Signs you're in freeze response:

- Unable to move
- Feeling disconnected and detached from thoughts and feelings
- Numbness
- Helplessness
- Stiffness or heaviness

Notice that these are all symptoms of depression.

Fear Responses

When we are very frightened or overwhelmed, our adrenalin and cortisol spike, which can trigger different fear responses. The purpose of these fear responses is keeping us safe from danger and, if they work, our body might trigger them the next time we get scared. The way we respond to stress in early life shapes which fear responses we'll use as adults.

There are five main fear responses that have been observed:

- **Fight – physically or verbally attacking the source of the threat.**
- **Flight – retreating either physically (running or hiding) or emotionally (switching off, avoiding, changing conversations).**
- **Freeze – becoming still and quiet (like playing dead). This occurs both physically (becoming immobile, unable to move or speak) and mentally (dissociating, numbing yourself).**
- **Flop – going floppy, which can involve physical illness and exhaustion.**
- **Fawn – trying to please the threatening person to stop them causing more harm; complying to minimise their upset or aggression.**

This can be a one-off experience – someone shouts at you, or you get into an accident. Or, if the threat is ongoing, the body can get stuck in freeze response and it can become a permanent state, often when there has been trauma in the past or you're experiencing chronic stress or highly emotional situations.

The idea that we have a 'window of tolerance' for these feelings was developed by professor of psychiatry Dr Daniel J. Siegel, in his 1999 book *The Developing Mind*, to illustrate our different responses to being overwhelmed. We all have a window of 'optimal arousal', where we're able to function well and manage our emotions. People who have faced trauma tend to have a narrower window of tolerance, so they shift into either hyper- or hypo-arousal more easily.

Hyperarousal is a heightened state of arousal that might feel like high anxiety, fear or anger. This triggers the fight-or-flight fear responses – it's all about doing, whether that's running or fighting. When you're hyper-aroused, it might feel hard to control your emotions and you might find it difficult to soothe or switch off.

Hypoarousal is a shutting-down of feelings, akin to the freeze or flop states. Your nervous system thinks it's helping you by shutting you down, cutting you off from pain. Unfortunately, it's actually creating severe disconnection from yourself and others.

These two states can be triggered by anything that feels threatening, or a feeling associated with past trauma. For George, it was his wife's pregnancy that conjured memories of the past and triggered his hypoarousal.

Tips to get out of the freeze response if you struggle with depression or disconnection

- **Get curious.** Identify your triggers. Try to think about areas of your life that bring high stress or are emotionally draining. What are the patterns or behaviours that tend to make you feel worse? By being curious about what might be triggering these feelings, you can start to become more aware of where the root cause might be.

- **Understand.** Are there any feelings, thoughts or memories in your life you're aware you're shoving into the dirty clothes cupboard, which probably need to be looked at? Start to understand exactly what you might be avoiding, and why.

- **Feel.** Connect to your body. Notice what you're feeling, any sensations you're aware of.

- **Act.** Move. Getting out of the freeze response is about moving and expressing the feelings to show your brain it's now safe. By consciously moving your body, you're sending signals to your brain that it's safe to move, it's safe to feel. This is an important part of regulating your nervous system. I'll give you more practical tools for this later (see page 89), as finding strategies to calm and soothe yourself can really help you to feel safe so you tolerate more feelings.

- **Repeat.** As with everything, this is not a one-time fix. Your body will likely go back into this fear response over and over. Be patient with yourself, this is a coping mechanism you would have developed because it once helped you survive something difficult. Just keep noticing when it happens and working the steps to try to feel safe again.

ANXIETY

Why Am I Anxious?

Kelley starts talking and doesn't stop for the full fifty minutes. As she speaks, I'm distracted by her movements. She's wearing leggings and a lace vest with a loose strap that keeps sliding off her shoulder. Her hair is in a blonde pineapple atop her head with strands around her face that she rearranges as she talks. It's often like this in a first session – the story people desperately want to be heard is on their lips, yearning to finally come out. The problem with Kelley is that, even as we settle into our work together, the talking does not let up. She starts the moment I open the door and doesn't come up for air until I shut it. While very common in the initial sessions, when the talking doesn't stop it can make the sessions difficult because I don't have space to speak. I have to fight to be heard, interrupting her mid-sentence. All the talking stops me from thinking, and I imagine it's keeping her from doing the same.

The issue, she tells me, is that she's overwhelmed. It's like she's at boiling point, constantly on the precipice of a panic attack. 'I'm too sensitive,' she tells me. 'I feel everything. It's like I don't have a skin, and everything gets into me.'

Her anxious thoughts span every element of her life. She has a constant sense of dread that something terrible is about to happen. She won't answer her phone in case it's someone ringing with bad news. She won't get on a plane, convinced it will crash, and every headache she has is a brain tumour. She replays situations over and over again, worries whether she said something stupid, whether people like her, whether people are mad at her.

I ask how long she's struggled like this. She says she was always an anxious kid, but it's got worse since she finished university. Transitions are a common time for anxiety to come up, whether it's ending university, moving house, changing jobs, ending a relationship, divorce, having kids, adult kids moving out; anything that destabilises your sense of security and brings uncertainty can trigger anxiety.

With no post-graduate job or sense of what she wants to do, the future of possibilities is terrifying to her. She's wants to be an artist but doesn't even know where to begin. She's confronted with option upon option, and has no idea how to figure out what she wants to do. Everything is a dilemma with a catastrophic end. What if she tries to make it in the art world and fails? What if she applies for a job and doesn't get it? What if she gets a job but ends up hating it? Maybe she should take a year out, but then she'll fall behind all her friends, and what if she can't afford to move out of her mum's house? Maybe she should move to a different country, but what if she hates that? Her dating life is much the same; each session she brings dating dilemmas that are more chaotic than the previous week's. Should she text her back? Is this girl even right for her? Is Kelley missing red flags?

I (as you might also be) am feeling exhausted just listening to Kelley's ruminations. It's hard to stay on one topic – she changes the subject, readjusts her hair, twists the rings on her fingers. I struggle to stay calm and grounded with this effervescing ball of nerves in front of me. At the same time, I'm really empathising with how much agony she's in – a reminder of just how crippling anxiety can be.

Why do we have anxiety?

It's very normal to feel anxious, especially in this uncertain world we live in. A little anxiety is even helpful – it's our survival system telling us that something might be dangerous and needs our attention. But many of us feel anxious all the time. It feels like the anxiety is eating us up, taking over our bodies and giving us no space to be anything other than a frantic ball of nerves.

Anxiety can take many forms: ruminating thoughts, worries about health, anxiety about relationships, fears of what other people think of us, obsessive thinking or behaviour, catastrophising, and a general sense of disquiet and dread. However it presents for you, it's important to listen to your anxiety, because it's telling you that something isn't quite right.

Symptoms of anxiety usually have a root that we're not aware of, and this root will be different for everyone. For some, anxiety will be a consequence of trauma – we never quite feel safe; we're hypervigilant and sensitive to things going wrong again; our nervous system is on high alert. For others, anxiety might have more of a relational root – we might feel socially anxious because we feel inferior to others; maybe we have anxiety around relationships because we fear being rejected and need to feel chosen. Or it might come from how we see ourselves – perhaps you're anxious about exams or work because deep down you don't feel good enough. It can also be a combination of many different things, a melting pot creating a sense of unease.

Can you see that the anxiety itself isn't the problem? It's a signpost that there's something under the surface. Rather than trying to get rid of anxiety, we need to understand what it is trying to tell us.

The catastrophe that's already happened

Anxious thoughts like Kelley's – that something bad is going to happen – generally stem from past experiences. Somewhere, at some point, it's likely something bad really did happen. For instance, in a review of studies on depression and anxiety, childhood trauma was shown to be one of the most significant risk factors for anxiety disorders, with exposure to trauma associated with a three to four times increased risk of depression and anxiety.[5]

We project the memories of the past onto the future to protect us from them happening again. Fear of being hurt, getting into trouble or being abandoned usually come from past experiences of these things happening. If you fear rejection, for example, it's likely because you've felt rejected before. People who haven't faced abandonment don't tend to fear it as much. So the root of the anxiety is usually coming from the helplessness you felt in the past.

We need to listen to this anxiety. It's pointing to a story from our past that requires attention. By talking about and processing the past, we can relocate the fears we're projecting onto the future back where they belong, freeing ourselves up for a more creative and hopeful future that is less frightening.

It might not always be a specific event that's causing the anxiety – a sense of instability can be more subtle than a one-off trauma. It could be that you grew up with unstable parents who struggled with anxiety themselves, maybe passing on their worries that the world isn't a safe place. If you didn't get enough emotional security, you might have a feeling of unsafety, that if something bad does happen you won't be protected. This can leave us feeling vulnerable and exposed, which is where the anxiety comes in. By worrying and obsessing, our minds feel a little more in control, which eases us from the terror of feeling insecure.

Staying in control

Imagine you're going about your day, feeling calm and content, when your friend sends you a slightly curt text. You panic. What have you done wrong? Are they angry with you? What do you reply? Do they hate you? You trail back through every possible thing that might have upset them. You're supposed to see them next week and now you're playing through every scenario that could happen, whether they're going to be off with you, what you can say to make them like you again.

By obsessing over what to reply, it makes us feel like we can control the other person's feelings about us. We cannot, of course, though this doesn't stop us trying.

Because we need relationships to survive, being rejected can feel – in a bodily sense – like a threat to our lives. So many of us are afraid of being disliked; we take everything personally and try desperately to control people's perceptions of us.

One of the key ways to ease anxiety is to accept the things we can't control. Fundamentally, if you can let go of control, anxiety can lessen. Kelley's anxiety keeps her feeling in control. Her catastrophising about the future is, in a way, an attempt to manage the fear of the unknown. If she can learn to accept that she cannot change or control the future, she might be able to soothe that anxious part of herself a little better.

Anxiety blocks feelings

Sometimes we get anxious because it's safer to feel anxiety than anything else. When we're anxious, it completely overtakes us; our hands start to sweat, our legs might shake, our throat goes dry, our thoughts race, our body rushes, we might struggle to sleep or eat or talk about anything other than the thing we're worried about.

If you were taught not to have certain feelings and you had parents who couldn't acknowledge your hurt and soothe you properly, you might unconsciously believe you shouldn't show certain feelings. Each time that feeling gets triggered, the real emotion is pushed down and instead we are flooded with anxiety for feeling that way at all.

However, even though anxiety can feel very big and alive, it is not a core feeling. In fact, anxiety totally blocks our body, so we don't sense any of our other feelings.

Now you might be thinking, 'But I AM feeling! My problem is that I'm feeling too much.' This is exactly what Kelley felt too – and indeed she does feel a lot – but anxiety isn't necessarily the same as feeling.

Sometimes, overthinking and stressing is actually a way of keeping out something more painful. Even if it seems like you're having lots of big emotions all the time, there are often still things in your unconscious you aren't aware of – none of us are. Anxiety can be a mechanism to avoid the deeper and more difficult feelings or memories in our unconscious. For example, when a relationship ends we might be consumed by anxiety – constantly thinking, planning what to say, obsessing about that person – but this anxiety is a way to stop us from feeling the more painful emotions of loss, grief, anger and deep sadness.

What if I have too many feelings?

Kelley seems to be suffering from feeling too much. She cries easily, panics at the drop of a hat, is highly sensitive and often struggles to calm her overwhelming emotions. There's something that seems infantile about this part of her, like a child who can't be calmed. When people weren't always emotionally soothed as children, they might find they struggle to soothe themselves as adults. I wonder whether that child part in Kelley was never taught to soothe herself.

If our needs are largely met in childhood – we have parents who are consistent, calm and emotionally attuned – we'll probably learn strategies to calm ourselves down when our feelings get too much. However, if we have parents who aren't able to meet our needs, we might learn that people are unreliable, and those feelings are never quite soothed. This can leave a kind of constant anxiety.

We might also have parents who try too hard to meet our needs, so we don't learn resilience. One of my favourite psychoanalysts, Donald Winnicott[6], explained in his seminal book *Playing and Reality*, that kids need a balance between having their needs met and being able to bear a little frustration at not having everything immediately. If they can learn to survive being overwhelmed by their uncomfortable feelings, just for a short while before their parents attend to their needs, they learn how to soothe themselves.

If you never learnt to soothe yourself, it might feel like you're a prisoner to your emotions and mood swings. A big part of the work of therapy is learning how to soothe yourself, how to tolerate discomfort and regulate your feelings – we'll talk about this more in Chapter 3 (see page 75).

Generally, what the anxiety is telling us is that something doesn't quite feel safe. Where that lack of safety comes from isn't always clear – maybe you grew up in an area where you were exposed to violence; maybe your parents fought a lot, which scared you as a child; maybe your parents had their own mental health struggles, or are part of a marginalised group that has been made to feel unsafe. Whether it's coming from your family, friends or society, the anxiety is a clue that somewhere in you there is a child who doesn't quite feel safe in the world.

For Kelley, I start to suspect that her anxiety is being exacerbated by poor boundaries. When you live in the world without strong boundaries, the world can feel very unsafe and out of control, which only feeds the anxiety.

Boundaries

A boundary is something that indicates a limit; it is a personal line drawn between you and another person. Boundaries define who we are, what we allow and what we don't. People speak a lot about boundaries because they are what keep us safe, they stop us from being used by others. Without boundaries we are completely at the mercy of others, feeling out of control and anxious. If you feel anxious about a situation, it might be a sign that you need to set a boundary to make yourself feel safe. Learning to put healthy boundaries in place can soothe our anxiety, by helping us to feel more empowered and in control.

Boundaries are taught to us as children. We may lack boundaries if our parents didn't have any. Lacking parental boundaries can look like:

- **Narcissistic parents who made us responsible for their feelings.**
- **Parents who put high expectations on us.**
- **Abuse, in which children's boundaries are violated by being exposed to sex or violence.**
- **Being made to do things we didn't want to do.**
- **Having no rules, never being told no or having too much power.**
- **Having parents who didn't see their children as separate people with their own minds.**

What have boundaries got to do with anxiety?

Kelley's struggles with boundaries quickly come to the fore in therapy. She comes to sessions too early or too late, often forgets to pay her bill, incessantly asks me questions about myself as though she can't bear not to know everything about me or to have any mystery or difference between us.

Therapy is a very boundary-led world; you arrive and leave on time, the session is at the same time slot each week, the bill must be paid every month, focus is kept on the patient rather than me. It's done this way for a reason: boundaries keep people safe. It's comforting to know you'll go to the same session at the same time each week, that the therapist will always be there, that things are usually the same. It's a little like having a secure base in our early attachment relationships – when the therapy is reliable and consistent, it helps us to feel contained and held, so that we can break open and take more risks. When people test the boundaries, like Kelley, it usually means they haven't had boundaries modelled for them.

I ask her what boundaries were like for her at home. She laughs and says, 'What boundaries? Mum's my best friend,' she explains. 'It's like we are the same person.'

Kelley's mum was very anxious in the early years of Kelley's life. When her husband died just months after Kelley was born, she became preoccupied with making sure she was a good enough mum. It was a struggle on her own, and his death triggered her abandonment issues. Determined to prove herself, she became fixated on making sure Kelley liked her. In a sense, it worked: they were best friends, told each other everything, had no secrets between them.

While this *Gilmore Girls*-style mother–daughter relationship might sound idyllic, it had a shadow side too. There was no privacy. Her mum would open her bedroom door without knocking, walk into the bathroom while Kelley was on the toilet, make Kelley feel guilty if she asked for distance or space or expressed a need that was different from her mum's. Because her mum was so desperate to be close, and sensitive to abandonment, Kelley felt completely responsible for her mum's happiness. In the process, she lost her ability to say no, and a great anxiety developed. Then, creating even more anxiety, when Kelley was around eight, her mum started dating. She would come home from dates, curl up on the sofa with Kelley and, though Kelley was too young to properly understand, tell her all the details about her sex life as if they were teenagers.

When children are made to grow up too fast, it can cause serious anxiety because that is, in itself, a boundary violation – being exposed to adult ideas or being made to feel responsible for your parents' feelings. They may also become co-dependent in their adult relationships (see page 235). I wonder if this is what she means when she says, 'I don't have a skin.' Perhaps it feels like there is no barrier between her and her mum, no sense of privacy or boundary between them.

Now, in the therapy room, Kelley is doing the same with me – she's not respecting the boundaries of the therapy, probably because she was never taught how. We're going to go through boundary setting in depth in the co-dependency section (page 248), where you'll hear more about Kelley and how she learnt to heal her anxiety.

– EXERCISE –

Try to remember the last time you felt anxiety rise up in you.

Get curious. *Listen to your anxiety as a signal of a blocked feeling and get curious. To do this you have to find a way to suspend judgement. Rather than trying to fight it or get rid of it, try to listen to it with compassion, as if it were a young child trying to tell you what is wrong.*

Understand. *Anxiety is actually a signal that there is something else wanting to be felt. Instead of punishing ourselves when we feel anxious, we can see it as a helpful clue that there is a feeling below that we need to accept and allow.*

Feel. *Try to get to what might be under these feelings. What might have triggered them? Are there any other feelings or sensations going on? When you feel anxious, try to find a quiet place where you can shut your eyes and focus on your body. Scan down from head to toe. Where do you feel the anxiety? Can you imagine digging under it and seeing what else might be there? Are there any twitches of sadness, or pulses of anger? Maybe it's a flutter of excitement or fear? You could be feeling several of these things at the same time; maybe that's confusing, to be both excited and scared at the same time, or both angry and happy. It's very normal to have more than one feeling at the same time. Instead of judging it, just allow whatever you can feel to be there.*

Act. *How would you soothe yourself if you were a child? Rather than getting angry or frustrated with the anxiety, try to give* *yourself what you would need if you were a child feeling afraid. What could you do to make yourself feel safer? Are there any boundaries you can put in place with this situation that might make you feel more held?*

Our triggers are our teachers

Now, I'm not suggesting that all of you reading who struggle with anxiety will have had similar experiences to Kelley. Some of you may have had parents who were the opposite of Kelley's mum – cold and distant, or avoidant of their feelings – which created its own kind of anxiety. The reason for your anxiety will be unique to you. Healing anxiety is really about finding the reason, processing what's underneath it and then giving yourself what you need to feel safe.

So instead of trying to fight your anxiety, let's think about how to change your relationship with it. Anxiety is trying to protect you from getting hurt again. It's a sign that there might be boundaries you need to set, that you feel out of control or that there are areas of your past that need attention. It sounds like a cliché, but you have to learn to stop hating it. Your anxiety is the part of you that's trying to keep you from danger.

Try thanking it and reminding it that you're safe now, so it doesn't need to worry any more. Trying to get rid of the symptoms of anxiety doesn't tend to work because they are there for a reason; they're serving a purpose. So rather than trying to fight anxiety, try to understand it. Have compassion for it and let it know, politely, that it's not needed any more.

What helped Kelley?

As the months go by, Kelley starts to slow down. She begins to come in on time and pay me each month. She stops asking me so many personal questions. I first notice the change when she arrives on time, sits down, takes a big sigh and leans back in the chair. 'What shall we talk about today?' she asks cheerily. Usually, Kelley's anxious ruminations start before she even sits down. Today she is still, present, peaceful.

'You seem different,' I say.

She looks at me. 'Yeah, I feel weirdly calm.' She pauses. 'Is that wrong?'

I laugh. 'Now you're getting anxious about not feeling anxious.' She laughs too, and I register the lightness, the sense of play between us. Something in Kelley is shifting.

The first thing that seemed to help Kelley was changing her relationship with her anxiety. Instead of seeing it as this terrible affliction that she needed to be rid of, we started to pay attention to it, to listen to what it was trying to say. 'It's been around since I was little,' Kelley explained, 'when things were super unstable and my mum was really worried too. I'd think something bad was going to happen all the time just because my mum was always on edge.' I wondered if the anxiety Kelley developed was partially her mum's, and partially a voice she'd developed to feel safe when things felt scary. 'So it's trying to help me? The anxiety?' I nodded and Kelley's brow furrowed. This was a new thought, that the anxiety might be trying to protect her, rather than make her life miserable. It's just that in protecting her, it was now doing more harm than good.

Understanding why your anxiety is there is the first step to changing it. Rather than fighting it, blaming it or even hating it, you need to recognise it is a symptom of a frightened part of yourself, and give that part of yourself the compassion it needs to feel safe so it can lower its guard a little.

As we talked about Kelley's past, other feelings started to come through other than the anxiety that tended to dominate. She admitted she was often furious with her mum, though she felt her mum was too fragile to handle her anger. The lack of personal space, the neediness, the demands placed upon her, had all built up in Kelley over the years, as she had no safe place to express her frustrations. This anger was healthy; it enabled Kelley to start building some independence by expressing difference from her mum, setting boundaries for how often they had dinner together (dropping from every day to twice a week), what they talked about (ending conversations when she started to feel like her mum was offloading onto her about her dates) and the decisions she made (lovingly letting her mum know that she is an adult now, that she appreciates her concern but ultimately she is going to make her own decisions). Setting these boundaries in her life helped Kelley to feel in charge of her life, as if she was now in the driving seat. Feeling more in control of your life, rather than at the whim of someone else, builds your inner sense of confidence and strength. 'My skin feels a little thicker,' Kelley announced one day after deciding to apply for an art course that would mean moving out of her mum's house. 'I feel like I can handle more.'

In later sessions, when the calm days became more frequent than anxious days, Kelley came in with a question. 'I'm confused why this is working – like, I don't get therapy. I'm much calmer and less worried, but for the life of me I cannot figure out what it is that's helped.' I smiled. This is a common question, and one I've struggled with myself because what helps is a combination of many things; there is no one solution. If I had to say what helped Kelley, I'd say it was a combination of processing her feelings about the past, accepting what she cannot control in the present and finding as much stability (through learning to set boundaries and advocate for her needs) so the future didn't feel as scary.

And even then, pinning it down to one solution – feeling your feelings, setting boundaries or soothing your nervous system – misses one of the most important aspects, the almost magical quality that is difficult to put into words: the therapeutic relationship itself.

It's no coincidence that Kelley started to set boundaries in her life just as she started to get used to the boundaries of therapy. She hadn't had the experience of someone who can hold and bear her feelings before. This was new for her – a safe and reliable relationship with someone who didn't want to merge with her, who wasn't too fragile to bear her anger and fear, who supported her independence and modelled boundaries. I'm not trying to toot my own horn or take credit for the hard work Kelley did, but I know from my own therapy the value in experiencing a relationship with someone who can both emotionally hold you and help you feel safe like this, especially if you haven't had that before.

That's why there is no quick fix to healing, and why it's difficult to summarise in a few neat points – because what works is an experience of something different. We don't tend to get better overnight. There isn't this eureka moment where everything suddenly changes, and your anxiety disappears in a flash. Instead, healing looks more like a random good day, then a chain of bad days, then another good day . . . until one day you realise it's been ages since your last panic attack or bout of anxiety. Healing creeps up on you; it's gentle and without drama. And, of course, it doesn't mean you'll never get anxious ever again.

Kelley's anxiety hasn't completely disappeared – naturally it still rears its head at times of uncertainty and stress. But we know now that when her thoughts start to race and the panic rises up, it's a sign that she needs to slow down, reflect on what's going on in her life, pay attention to her feelings, adjust her boundaries and do what she can to find stability and soothe herself.

Tips for soothing anxiety in the moment

- **Ground yourself.** Do what you can to feel more in control – name items in the room, use your hands to make something, notice what you can hear and touch around you.

- **Breathe.** Make your out-breath longer than your in-breath, which relaxes your nervous system.

- **Tell someone.** Keeping it trapped inside can make it bigger. Telling someone safe how you're feeling can help to calm you in the moment.

- **Write.** Put all your anxious thoughts down so they aren't going round and round your head. With no filter, just let yourself freely express.

- **Move.** Release the energy physically through your body – go for a walk, dance around your room, go boxing, scream into a pillow. Try to give space to your feelings by expressing them however your body wants to move.

- **Reflect.** Once you're calmer, try to think about what might have triggered you, and whether there are any other feelings being masked by the anxiety.

These tools might help in the moment, but they won't necessarily prevent the anxiety from coming back again. They are techniques for dealing with the tip of the iceberg – they are helpful in the moment, but to really reduce your anxiety long-term, you need to get underneath.

TRAUMA, STRESS AND THE NERVOUS SYSTEM

Why Can't I Relax and How Do I Heal from Trauma?

The clock ticks. A tiny light blinks in the corner of the ceiling. An engine rattles somewhere. Footsteps from a neighbour using the bathroom. A siren just close enough to hear. Arlon sighs audibly. He dares himself to look at the clock. Four in the morning. He sighs again, more of a growl this time, and flips over on his side. Sleep has yet to come, for five nights in a row.

As the room fills with light, the consequences of another sleepless night fill his body. Head throbbing, eyes heavy, limbs leaden. His mood suffers more; he feels depressed and irritable and close to tears.

The lack of sleep wreaks havoc on his immune system. He gets run down with colds most weeks, random rashes appear without invitation, headaches strike him at inopportune moments, often during busy periods at work when he can't afford to take time off. He's sluggish and in pain, almost constantly sick and never quite feels well enough to give 100 per cent to anything.

Everything in Arlon's life would be fine if it weren't for his body trying to betray him.

He searches for the answers to what's wrong. Bouncing from GPs to specialists, he finds himself in a revolving door of doctor's appointments, walking out with new prescriptions to fight problems he can't pronounce. They diagnose him with adrenal fatigue, a vitamin deficiency, gut microbiome imbalance, various allergies. Just as he tackles one symptom, another pop ups like a game of Whac-a-Mole.

He suffers through his days, confused and unclear about what's wrong.

During one of the dark stretches of reluctant wakefulness, he listens to a podcast about stress and physical health. Desperate to feel better, he impulsively books a therapy appointment. One session can't hurt. As the date approaches, anxiety creeps through in the form of a list of reasons why therapy won't work. Ten minutes before the session, he cancels. He's not the type of person to go to therapy – he doesn't need that kind of help. Besides, this is a physical issue, so what good will it do to talk about things? He needs solutions, not talking.

He spends another year in search of the answer, only growing sicker and more stressed. The headaches get stronger and more frequent. He gets some form of flu most weeks. He barely sleeps, waking with red eyes and a sour mind. Finally, after he's tried everything, his partner convinces him to give therapy a go again. Too exhausted to fight, he relents. What has he got to lose?

How does stress make us sick?

Have you found yourself coughing and spluttering, unable to get out of bed right after a stressful period in your life? Maybe you were working hard, burning the candle at both ends, not sleeping well, and you found yourself coming down with the flu. It's like your body is saying to you, 'No more, we need rest and recovery now.' Everyone's body will be different: some will get severe headaches, bad sleep, maybe stomach aches and gut issues. Your body is communicating something to you – that it needs a break.

What happens when this stress is constant? When our bodies have been stressed for years and a few days in bed isn't enough to calm us down? Constant stress in the body can lead to more chronic conditions, like autoimmune disorders, cancer, diabetes, heart attack and stroke.

Everything that's ever happened to us lives in our body, whether it's positive or negative, whether we remember it or not. Our body is the constant vessel that experiences everything we go through. As we live our lives, our bodies are constantly adapting for survival.

You've read so far that when things are too traumatic, our mind and body separate, and all the difficult parts can get repressed into the unconscious. While our mind might forget our negative experiences, our bodies do not. You might feel completely at ease in your mind, as if the past didn't affect you at all, but your body tells a different story.

Are you stuck in the fear response?

In his bestselling book *The Body Keeps the Score*, psychiatrist Bessel van der Kolk[7] goes into detail about the effects of trauma on the body as well as a whole range of different treatments to help it heal.

He explains that trauma is essentially a big shock to the system. When we're afraid, our body will activate the fear response – fight, flight, flop or fawn – and secrete adrenaline, cortisol and other stress hormones.

To release this shock and come out of the fear response, emotions need to be processed. However, when that shock doesn't get released – which it often doesn't for humans – it stays trapped in the body and unconscious, so your nervous system gets stuck in fear mode. If you weren't given space to process your feelings after the trauma, they don't get released from your body and your nervous system stays in a heightened state.

When you're stuck in this constant state of fear and alertness, you don't know the difference between a real threat and a perceived threat, so, like an oversensitive fire alarm, your nervous system sounds off at any slight notion of danger, releasing all the stress hormones and triggering that fear response all over again. Traumatised people might overreact to loud noises or be very sensitive to other people's moods. They might never feel relaxed, find it hard to be still or be jumpy and hypervigilant because their nervous system is stuck in a fear state, ready for something bad to happen again.

Why don't humans complete the stress cycle easily?

Did you know that when prey animals like antelopes have been chased by lions and managed to escape, their entire body shakes in fear of what's just happened. In Dr Peter Levine's book *Waking the Tiger: Healing Trauma*[8], he noticed that wild animals don't tend to suffer from dysregulated nervous systems in the same way as humans. He realised that the antelopes shake to release all the adrenaline and stress hormones from the shock. After the shaking is over and the stress hormones have been discharged, the antelope simply hops back up, dusts itself off and continues like nothing has happened. The stress cycle has been completed.

For humans, it's not so simple. We bury our feelings if they can't be spoken about or expressed, because we're so afraid they'll cause us to be rejected – especially if our parents weren't attuned to our feelings or good at regulating themselves.

When we're young, we're so much more vulnerable and dependent upon others to feel safe. So, if traumas occur when we're young and we don't have a nurturing caregiver who can soothe us, our nervous system might stay in fear mode for most of our adult life.

We might not even realise we're in fear mode because it's become so normal that we don't notice it, so here are some key signs that your nervous system is dysregulated.

Symptoms of a dysregulated nervous system

- Difficulty falling asleep or staying asleep.
- Headaches.
- Autoimmune problems.
- Gut and digestive issues.
- Impaired memory.
- Never feeling relaxed.
- Anxiety and panic attacks.
- Chronic fatigue.

- Explosive anger.
- Low self-worth.
- Difficulty self-soothing.
- Skin problems and inflammation.
- Addiction.
- Eating disorders.
- Feeling emotionally numb or dissociated.
- Not being able to be still.
- Chronic pain.
- Catastrophising.
- Frequently getting ill.
- Hypervigilance – being jumpy or overly sensitive to loud sounds.

If you experience any of these, with no clear physical reasons as to why, it could be a sign that your body is more stressed than you realise. Often, physical health problems are a sign that the body is expressing what the mind cannot. Being stuck in the stress response impacts our immune system, which can stop us from being able to fight off disease. There are countless studies showing the link between high stress, trauma and physical health problems such as cancer, diabetes, heart attack and stroke, autoimmune disorders, gut issues, sleep problems and more.[9] Even if you don't realise you are stressed or have faced any traumas, your body might be telling you something you don't want to hear. So, rather than ignoring it, try to listen to what it might be trying to say.

Attachment and the Nervous System

Not all stressed nervous systems are caused by a single traumatic event, such as a car crash, or being hit or shouted at; there can also be consequences on the nervous system from attachment styles (see page 211). Safe relationships are essential to protect children, as they aren't able to regulate themselves in the early years. When parents are good enough, co-regulation can take place, where they will help children to regulate their emotional states, so they are able to soothe themselves as adults. Insecure attachment relationships can lead to inadequate co-regulation of the nervous system, resulting in a dysregulated nervous system as an adult.

This is especially true if the parents are a cause of the stress. When the usual response to stress – to turn to your caregiver – isn't possible, children don't find a way to regulate their own feelings without turning to external tools (such as food, dissociation, repression, avoidance, being overly emotional). Because children are still developing, inadequate regulation at this age can have significant consequences on the brain, the nervous system and physical health.

Arlon's nervous system

I first realise just how fearful Arlon is in one of our earlier sessions. He's talking about a situation at work. He was giving a presentation to a client when he started to feel a migraine coming on. As the edges of his vision blurred, he tried to continue, praying they didn't notice how the sweat was pooling at his armpits or the way he winced at every word. As he tells me about the punishing look from his boss, my doorbell rings. Arlon is startled. He takes a sharp breath and sits upright. The colour drains from his cheeks. It's as if a lion has roared or a bomb has gone off. He looks at me with wide pupils, like a child watching for reassurance that everything's going to be OK.

'Sorry about that.' I try to speak gently, to soothe his terror. 'It seems like that frightened you.'

'It's fine,' he says – a polite version of back the hell off. I respect his defences and wait. His bottom lip quivers. 'I think I've been scared my whole life.'

Now, it might seem that these two things are unrelated – Arlon's jumpiness and his physical health problems – but my guess is that Arlon may have faced some trauma that has made him chronically afraid (i.e. he has a dysregulated nervous system), which might be why he's so often unwell.

So I try to understand what might have happened that made Arlon so afraid in the first place.

Why do we get stuck in the fear response?

We might think of this kind of jumpiness as being a form of post-traumatic stress disorder (PTSD) someone develops after going to war, being in a crash or being abused. While these events are indeed traumatic, we know now that there are different levels of trauma. Your nervous system can become dysregulated as a result of both big-T trauma and little-t trauma. The fear response will be more severe in people who have experienced sexual, physical or emotional abuse or neglect, but your nervous system can still be dysregulated by small-t traumas.

Children can be traumatised by any experience in which their needs are not being met, which, if not properly processed, can create an overactive fear response. You might not even clearly remember anything bad happening to you at an early age, but your body likely will.

Having a parent whose own nervous system is dysregulated can also cause our nervous system to become dysregulated. Maybe one of your parents is anxious or angry or traumatised themselves. Even if you didn't experience obvious trauma, being raised by someone whose nervous system is on high alert can stop you from learning to soothe yourself and feel relaxed, so you too stay on high alert. They're teaching you, through the way they react to things, that the world is not a safe place.

– EXERCISE –

1. *Notice what's going on in your body. Take a deep breath and just be aware of any sensations.*

2. *Ground yourself in safety. Can you think of a time when you felt calm and safe? Remember how that felt in your body.*

Picture yourself there, completely relaxed and carefree, and come back to this whenever you need to ground yourself.

3. *Think of a time when you felt stress. It doesn't have to be a big trauma. Let's start with something small. How did it feel to be stressed? Where did you notice it? What's your body doing now as you remember it? Are there any changes in your body from the calm state? Allow whatever feelings are there to come up. If you want to cry, cry; if you want to scream, scream; let your body do whatever it wants. Are there any images or words that come up? Notice it all without judgement.*

4. *Once you feel ready, go back to your safe, grounded place. Notice how your body changes. Can you feel yourself relax? What shifts happen in your breathing, chest or other areas of tension? Take your time, and let your body come to a calm state.*

This exercise is a first step in going from stress to safety. By allowing yourself to process the feelings from the stressful event, you're releasing those stress hormones – like the antelope shaking – and then allowing your body to return to safety and calm.

This kind of exercise can be used after any stressful event to help you process it in the moment so it doesn't leave your body stuck in the fear response. It can also be used to process traumatic events, but I would encourage you to do this with a professional who can help you to really feel secure and process the trauma slowly and safely.

How Arlon started to heal

After learning about the fear response, Arlon realises that his nervous system has been on high alert his whole life. Sleep for Arlon is dangerous. It's the time when he is most vulnerable and cannot protect himself. Together we realise that his body won't let him sleep because it needs to keep one eye open on what might go wrong.

His healing process is multilayered. We talk about the scary things that happened to him when he was a child. The way he'd walk on eggshells around his stepdad, trying to say and do all the right things so as not to anger him. The way his heart would fall into his stomach when he heard tyres on the gravel. The way he'd pull the covers over his head, trying to block out the crashing of glass and the cries from his mother downstairs.

We work on helping his mind and body learn that he is no longer in danger. First, it's important he tells his story. This is partly because he's never talked about himself in a reflective way before, and partly because we need to build a sense of safety between us before he can start to connect his story to the difficult feelings in his body. Then we start to work on him connecting to his body. Each session I ask what's going on in his body, how he feels and where any tension is. At the beginning it's hard – he mostly just feels anxious and jumpy, unable to stay with a feeling for long – but as time goes on it gets a little easier. He starts to notice a fear in the back of his neck, a sense of panic fizzing in his fingers. He also notices pleasant sensations too: a warm glow in his chest or the grounding comfort of his back against the chair.

As he comes to connect more to his body, he starts to carry this outside of the therapy room too. He uses a mindfulness app and joins a breathwork group where he spends an hour a week focusing on his breath and relaxing into his body. After those sessions he finds he sleeps a little deeper. Throughout the day he naturally checks in with his body more, noticing when he feels more stressed and on edge, compared to when he feels relaxed.

After what he calls the 'fizzy' days, he makes a conscious effort to come home and do some deep breathing or go for a gentle walk to calm himself down. He notices the fizzing at work too. When things are really fizzy and he becomes totally overwhelmed, he takes five minutes to breathe deeply in the toilets or goes for a stroll around the block.

It isn't a miracle cure straight away. He comes to therapy with a throbbing head after a week of sleepless nights, frustrated that all this effort is amounting to nothing. 'I know it's frustrating,' I say, 'but you've been scared for your whole life – give it time.' He perseveres, and slowly, without either of us really noticing, he starts to improve. He sleeps a full eight hours for the first time in years.

How do you heal trauma?

First, it's important for you to know that profound healing from trauma is possible. Processing trauma can have life-changing consequences for people. This doesn't mean you'll be completely free of the effects of trauma. The reality is, we cannot undo trauma, but we can find a way to live well with it.

People often ask me how to heal trauma, and how long it will take. It's hard to give a clear answer because healing is multifaceted, and different things work for different people. Everyone who experiences trauma will respond differently to triggers and treatments. Even for one person, no one treatment alone will be the answer – healing is often a combination of different mind and body practices together.

The first step is to acknowledge that trauma has happened. If this word feels too strong for what you've experienced, you can call it something else. Maybe some of your needs weren't met as a child. The important thing is to recognise that the past has affected you.

Then the aim is to make it safe to be in your body and tolerate your buried feelings. By connecting to the feelings and memories that are trapped in your body, you can release them. To come out of the fear response that your nervous system is stuck in, your body has to learn that it is now safe, that the danger from the past is over. This can reverse the split between your mind and body, verbalising what's happened to you as a way to reintegrate the feelings that have been cut off.

Even if you don't consciously remember an event, your body might remember. By noticing the sensations in your body and allowing whatever feelings are coming up, you can start to release the trauma.

While it can be really helpful to make meaning of the things that have happened to us, talking alone is not enough. To really process trauma you have to physically connect with it. Talking about a trauma without connecting to the feelings doesn't always help, because it's the unconscious feelings that have been trapped in the body that you're trying to release.

In *The Body Keeps the Score*, Bessel van der Kolk writes that the body needs 'experiences that deeply and viscerally contradict the helplessness, rage or collapse that result from trauma'.

When the repressed feelings can be experienced and nothing bad happens, your mind and body can learn that there is nothing to be afraid of any more and start to come out of the fear response.

Three golden rules for healing trauma

1. **Take your time.** Because you need to feel safe in order to really connect to the emotional pain, this process can take time. It is not something that should be rushed. The priority is to make sure you feel safe and don't get too overwhelmed. It might mean you have to go over things repeatedly, but each time you do you might get a little deeper and connect to the feelings a little more.

2. **Don't retraumatise.** It can be traumatising to go back over the exact details of the things that have happened, overwhelming the nervous system all over again as if the traumas are happening again. Processing is less about replaying the traumatic things that have happened, and more about allowing whatever feelings or images from the past rise up. Often, it's not about going over and over past events; instead, you might be triggered by something that's happening in your present life. Rather than going back through the trauma, we can work with the feelings that are coming up in the here and now.

3. **Ask for help.** This isn't something that's easy to do alone. While you are the only one who can really heal you, it can be so healing to have a witness to experience it with you and help you feel safe. Often, we've buried the feelings because we've learnt it's not safe to be vulnerable with someone else. It's the very act of connecting to those feelings in the presence of another that can help us to feel safe again.

Tips to feel safe in your body

- **Co-regulation.** In therapy, sitting with someone who can witness your pain as well as hold and contain it can really help to soothe your nervous system. By seeing that the therapist is OK, hasn't exploded or abandoned you for showing your vulnerability, your mind and body learns that these feelings are OK to have, that you don't need to feel so afraid any more. When children's feelings have been regulated by their parents they eventually learn to regulate on their own. If you've experienced trauma, you may never have learnt how to regulate. It's a similar process that happens in therapy when you co-regulate with the therapist, which gives you the tools to then soothe yourself.

- **Breathe.** Any slow mindfulness practices like yoga, breathwork or meditation can help soothe you and bring you out of that fear response. One proven way to calm your nervous system is to make your out-breath longer than your in-breath. Breathe in for four counts and breathe out for eight counts. Do this for ten minutes when you're stressed and see how much calmer you feel.

- **Move your body.** I don't mean exercise, though this has many benefits to your mental and physical health too; I mean moving your body to express the feelings. Maybe you want to shout, punch a pillow or scream into it. Maybe you want to be slow, hug yourself and show tenderness. Maybe you want to actually run to mimic the flight response. Whatever your body wants to do, let it move how it wants. Think of that antelope shaking to release the stress hormones. If you feel silly, that's OK – feeling silly is a small price to pay.

- **Touch and massage.** By getting to know your body again, touching yourself or allowing yourself to be touched by others, you're teaching it that it is safe to be in your body and encouraging it to relax into a more regulated, calm state. This can involve hugs from a safe partner, professional massages or self-touch where you hug or stroke yourself.

Finally, an important part of healing is recognising that we are never fully healed, and taking care of the wounded parts of ourselves by being compassionate and understanding to ourselves instead of self-critical. This might be recognising that in an overwhelming party we may need ten minutes of alone time, or not taking on too many stressful work commitments, rather than comparing ourselves unfavourably with people who seem to be able to manage these things easily. We might never be able to fully undo what's happened to us, but we can learn to accept it, and live differently with it.

ADDICTION
Why Can't I Stop?

The first thing Lana does after we sit down is take out her phone to send a quick email before we start. I'm feeling a little snubbed, but it gives me a chance to take her in – charcoal power suit, heels, scraped-back hair, concentrated frown on her face. The second thing she does is ask whether sessions can be thirty minutes, as opposed to the usual fifty. Work is busy right now and she's not sure she can give up a full hour of her time.

What is it that Lana is really telling me here? She's telling me work is more important than therapy, that this is not a priority, that she wants to control the boundaries of our time. Therapy often starts with a power struggle of this kind – sometimes people need to test your boundaries to make sure you're safe, that you're not going to keel over if pushed. While it sounds like it might be helpful to Lana to be accommodating, I get the sense that she's wanting me to let her know she's safe with me, that there are fixed boundaries here, that she can't run this show.

I tell her sessions are fifty minutes. She rolls her eyes but agrees to try to make the full session work – which I take as a sign that I've passed this first boundary test.

Then she tells me, explicitly, that she does not have a problem. She is health conscious, rarely drinks, has never smoked, exercises three times a week and is highly committed to her job. It's challenging being a woman in the male-dominated industry of law, but she's hard-working and now a highly esteemed barrister. People are scared of her, she tells me proudly. I get it. I, too, am a little scared of her. I don't say this, of course, but let her continue. Over the years the pressure has mounted up and work has become the sole focus in her life. Lana doesn't sleep much. She wakes at six to get to the office early and leaves around nine in the evening (if she's lucky). 'I'm here for Antony,' she explains. Her partner, Antony, feels she's neglecting him and their boys. He barely sees Lana; the kids ask why Mummy doesn't have dinner with them or ever come to watch one of their matches.

'I don't want to be a single father,' he tells her, 'but that's what it feels like.' He doesn't want to leave, though he might have no choice if she can't find a way to have better boundaries with work, so Lana is here, reluctantly, to save her marriage. She has no interest in working less.

The first time she's twenty minutes late I give her the benefit of the doubt. She couldn't get out of the meeting; it won't happen again. We have a thirty-minute session instead, just like she asked for at the beginning. The second and third time I still don't say anything, waiting to see if she settles into being on time. Then the fourth time it starts to feel like a pattern. A pattern in the therapy room is usually an unconscious communication of something. I'm just not sure what yet.

Like Antony, I start to feel neglected, as if she doesn't care about me or the therapy, and I start to question whether she really cares about herself. If her energy is poured into work, she doesn't have to think about herself. So, when she finally arrives, twenty minutes late, I ask her if she's uncomfortable having a full session, if she's trying to avoid something by being late. 'No,' she says, 'it's just that work takes priority.'

'Over you?' I ask. 'This is your time for yourself.'

She rolls her eyes. 'You sound just like Antony.'

This is not the classic picture of an addict, but addiction is really any compulsive behaviour used to manage psychological pain. Lana cannot stop working – I suspect because if she did, she'd have to feel the pain.

Nathan

In contrast, Nathan's addictions are more conventional. He's struggled with drugs and alcohol since he was fourteen. At first, he was just keeping up with everyone else, but now he's thirty-five and his friends are starting to settle down, he's realised he's the only one who still wants to party every weekend. His work is suffering, he's often hungover and he has embarrassed himself at one too many office parties. His partner recently broke up with him because they wanted someone more serious, less of a mess. Even his brother tried to stage an intervention.

Nathan first started drinking to fit in. There were boys in the year above who took a dislike to him because he was camp and effeminate. People spread rumours that he was gay before he even really understood what that meant. 'I was at an all-boys school in the nineties,' he told me. 'The word "gay" was a slur back then. No one wanted to have anything to do with me.' The bullying was subtle but insidious: sniggering when he walked into a room, moving desks as far away from him as possible, always picking him last for sports teams. His friends turned against him for fear of being condemned by association. Nathan spent most of his breaktimes alone and miserable.

One day, the ringleader and his followers snuck into the changing rooms while Nathan was showering after PE. It took all his might to suck in his tears as they laughed at him dripping in his towel as he hunted in panic for his clothes. Later, cowering in the headteacher's office in stained lost-property trackies, he promised himself he was not going to let this happen again. He needed to do something to impress them, to show them he was manly, acceptable, cool.

He came to school the next day with an offering – a bottle of rum from his dad's alcohol cabinet. They snuck sickly sweet sips round the back of the gym at lunchtime. He couldn't believe how his plan worked. One day he was being humiliated, the next he was drinking with the cool crowd. They wiped their mouths with their sleeves and stashed the empty bottle behind a tree. 'Can you get us another one?'

'Course.' Nathan nodded as if his life depended on it.

Paying his bottle tax each day, he started to be accepted by the group. He went from being beaten up and mocked to being invited to parties. The gay slurs stopped, and by the time he'd got to grips with his sexuality, he didn't dare come out for fear of what they might do. Instead, he drank. The wilder he acted, the more they approved. He was the drunkest at every party, the one to buy all his new friends fake IDs, the first to smoke weed and then take pills. Drinking was how he earned respect and power. Unfortunately, this was not a long-term solution. Now he's an adult, people no longer respect him. In fact, when he's the last one swaying in the bar as the lights come up, he can feel them looking at him the way they used to at school, like he's pathetic, a loser. Except Nathan cannot stop.

It is this that defines addiction – not the substance or the behaviour itself, but something that someone cannot stop. Why can't we stop? Why can't Lana just work less to save her relationship? Why can't Nathan quit drinking like everyone is telling him to? Why couldn't I stop eating?

We cannot stop because the addictive behaviour is serving an important purpose: it is keeping us from pain. Even though the addiction and the terrible consequences it might cause create potentially greater difficulties, our minds think that the original pain we're numbing ourselves from is more dangerous. By distracting and numbing our minds from the anxiety underneath, we're running from the unconscious truth we don't want to face.

What causes addiction?

To heal from addiction we have to understand what the emotional pain is and why we aren't able to soothe ourselves. Babies rely on their parents to learn to soothe themselves. A secure parent will teach their child that their feelings are manageable by being able to attune to what their baby needs and help soothe them. Much of this has nothing to do with words. A secure parent who responds to their child's needs will make a baby feel safe, which calms their nervous system and teaches them to regulate their feelings. If your parents were stressed or depressed themselves, absent, not emotionally literate or actively abusive, they may not have made you feel safe and calm. This leads us to find other ways to manage, through addictive behaviours that release pleasurable and rewarding hormones that make us feel, in the moment, soothed.

We're trying to fill a hole of care and attention that we didn't get. In his work on narcissism, psychologist Heinz Kohut talks about addiction and mental health in terms of deficits[10] – they are the result of deficits in early relationships. Substance use or other addictions are attempts to make up for the deficit, as if the thing we're addicted to is a pseudo mother we never had who soothes us and is always there.

Addiction

The reliance on any substance or behaviour to avoid difficult thoughts or feelings in our unconscious. You may not know the reason, or that there is something you're trying to avoid, but if you find yourself unable to stop doing any of the things mentioned below, chances are you're using them to cope with something you don't want to look at.

That's not to say that trauma that happens to us in adulthood can't trigger addiction – it absolutely can – but often those early relationships are what shape how we respond to difficult experiences as adults. If we have a deficit in care and emotional attention, we probably won't have developed the skills to regulate our emotions and care for ourselves in the healthiest way.

When we experience trauma and we don't have parents who are emotionally attuned enough to help us cope, life creates more pain than our young minds are able to process. Something happens that is profoundly difficult, and it is simply too much for us to bear. What happens when things are too much? Our mind and body, very cleverly, splits everything up into compartments. It takes all of those overwhelming feelings and sends them away, down into the unconscious where we don't have to feel them.

We aren't numb because we're empty, but because we are too full with pain. To numb that pain we turn to coping mechanisms, and they can take many forms . . .

A (non-exhaustive) list of behaviours used to cope with internal pain

- Over-exercising
- Disordered eating
- Buying things
- Social media
- Gambling
- Porn and/or masturbation
- Television
- Obsessive cleaning

- Sex and relationships
- Work
- Video games
- Drugs and alcohol
- Seeking conflict and drama
- Sugar (and overeating in general)
- Checking the news
- Obsessive thoughts or behaviours (OCD).

You might read this and notice that you do some of these things. Don't be alarmed. Distraction and numbing are perfectly normal, especially in the world we live in today.

The behaviour or substance itself in some ways does not really matter, though of course it will undoubtably change the severity of the troubles it creates in your life. A heroin addiction is a different beast to an addiction to exercise or television, but the root is the same – it's being used to keep darker feelings and thoughts away.

We think of these things as being self-destructive, and that's exactly right; we are trying to destroy a part of ourselves – the part that is vulnerable and wounded and terrified to be known.

What helped Lana?

Let's use our framework here to look at what helped Lana start to heal.

Get curious

Lana was only able to explore her work addiction once she admitted it was a problem for her (rather than for me or her husband). Yet again she was late to a session, and I started to get annoyed. Here I was, on time, ready to start and I had to sit twiddling my thumbs waiting for her to arrive, without even a courtesy text to let me know she'd be late. It's not only addicts who experience huge consequences from their behaviour; it's often the case that other people in their lives also suffer, and therefore have to hold the problem – first Antony and now me. I wanted Lana to own that it was a problem, rather than holding it for her.

When she finally walks through the door, I set a hard boundary. 'Lana,' I say, 'your lateness is depriving you of your full session time. Maybe we need to think together about whether therapy is something you are able to commit to.' It was a risk – I didn't want to stop working with Lana, but I also needed her to experience the consequences rather than me.

She looked at me with a furious stare, then her face crumpled, and with it her whole body into a heap of relief. 'You're right,' she said, 'I can't commit. I can't commit to anything. Work is ruining my relationship, now it's ruining this – it's ruining my life.' I breathed a syrupy sigh of relief, and so did she. It's hard work to maintain those defences. I could see that in admitting the problem something had been released for Lana. 'Why am I like this?' she asked, her vulnerability coming through.

'I don't know,' I said. 'Let's try and find out together.'

Understand

Lana comes in flustered but on time. She's less put-together than normal – there's a sense of anxiety about her I haven't seen before.

'I had a weird dream last night,' she says, fast. 'There was this leak in a boat and water was flooding in. I was trying to patch it up, fill it with whatever I could find, but this guy kept coming and taking it all out, and I'd try to shove more stuff in, then I got really annoyed because the water was getting higher and higher and so I shouted at this man, "What are you doing?" and I looked up and it was Jack.'

'Jack?' I say. 'Who's Jack?'

'Er, no one.' She pauses. 'I have an uncle, Jack,' Lana says, trailing off. I try to meet her eye, to show my confusion; she stares at the wall, eyes vacant, as if she's been taken over by a spirit or has simply left her body. She says nothing. I have the urge to wave in front of her face, to bring her back to life. She continues to gaze into space as the words come out.

'Uncle Jack,' she says to the wall, 'he wasn't a good person.' She shakes her head and comes to, meeting my eyes once more. 'I don't want to talk about that, is that all right?'

I nod carefully, knowing that Lana needs to feel safe in this moment but that eventually we might need to come back here.

She misses the next two sessions – work obligations, apparently – then arrives on time, nervous and ready to tell her story.

Both Lana's parents worked late nights, so Uncle Jack would pick her up from school, get her fed and put her to bed. She doesn't remember much – her memories have been mostly blacked out – but she knows he used to touch her. Her eyes flick to me, checking this is OK. I nod, realising how important this is for her to put into words. She didn't tell anyone; she was too young to know what was even happening, never mind how to speak about it. All she knew was that it was wrong. So she started to stay later at school, buying time before she'd have to go home to Uncle Jack. She'd take on extra homework, revise intently for every exam, join after-school clubs and sometimes, when everything was completed, she'd even invent work to do – anything to avoid going home.

Work was soothing for her; it was safe, free from danger. As an adult, she continues to toil away, though she's lost touch with what she's even working so hard for.

Putting words to a story that is unspeakable is profoundly important. Of course, we can't always make meaning from the things that have happened to us. There is no sense to sexual abuse, no greater meaning. Sometimes horrible things happen without rhyme or reason. But what we can do is try to find the words to express the horrors that live within our bodies.

Talking is such an important part of reshaping traumatic experiences – making sense of the things that have happened to us and telling the stories that have been locked inside us for years. Honestly, this is one of the greatest privileges of my job. Nothing is more moving than sitting with someone who is telling their story for the first time, or seeing it in a new way. For Lana, putting words to this unspeakable thing made what happened a little more bearable, and helped her to lessen the shame she'd been carrying all these years.

Feel

As we put words to what happened to Lana, the feelings come tumbling through. She sobs, she yells, she whimpers, she even sometimes laughs. They have to be slowly teased out at first; it's very uncomfortable for Lana to admit she was in the least bit vulnerable. I once thought that too, and I learnt, over a long time, that I am vulnerable, and so are you. We all are, whether we're feeling it or not.

As we talk more about her past, and how she operates in her present, Lana comes to realise that work is helping her run not only from the past, but also from her current relationship. She notices that she became busier when she and her partner grew closer. 'What is it you're scared of?' I ask.

'I don't know,' she says. 'That he'll see I care, that if I let myself need him, he'll stop caring or something and it will hurt even more.' It seems that Lana is also addicted to work as a way to avoid having to feel dependent upon her husband, and to numb the pain and fear of not feeling cared about.

Act

Lana starts to acknowledge how fearful she is of depending on Antony. To protect herself from the sexual abuse, she stopped letting herself get close to anyone, especially men. Work was serving as an escape. Together we concoct a plan – when she gets the urge to take on more work or cancel plans with Antony to work, it is probably a sign that underneath she is scared and feeling the need to protect or soothe herself. It takes a long time, a few failed attempts and a lot of drafts in her Notes app, but eventually she tells Antony about her past, and why she's been so focused on work all these years. They both cry, and he holds her, promising he won't hurt her. As she starts to speak her fears, the need to work lessens. She sets boundaries with her team and reduces her hours to make more time for pleasure in her life. The purpose work was serving (to run away from herself and her relationship) is no longer needed.

Repeat

For the purposes of the story, this might seem like a linear process, but believe me it is not. Lana would get curious, understand something and feel it, then she'd go back to saying she was fine and didn't feel anything, work late again and cancel a session. Then there would be another chink in the armour, she'd show some vulnerability, have a cry and maybe it would translate into action. Then she'd come in the next week twenty minutes late again, back at square one, saying that the therapy isn't working and she doesn't have a problem. It was like Lana was a frightened turtle, daring to stick her head out for a moment, then immediately retreating into her shell of safety. After a while, she'd stick her head out a little further, and then hide all over again. The process is one of pauses and back-steps, because that's what people have to do to feel safe. But this is part of the magic of it, because with each repetition, another layer is processed. And eventually, Lana was able to step out of her shell safely and live a different kind of life.

So how do I heal?

As a therapist, I try to talk little of the actual addiction or distraction, much to my patients' dismay (the addiction is often the only thing they want to talk about), and instead I try to steer the conversation towards the thing they don't want to talk about: the pain they're numbing.

Tackling the addiction, trying to quit, exercising willpower and creating better habits are useful pursuits, but they are the tip of the iceberg and are unlikely to really heal the root of the addiction. When we describe ourselves or others as someone with an addictive personality, we are really describing a person who is sensitive or traumatised and trying to regulate their difficult feelings. You can try to take away the substance or behaviour, but the need to soothe will persist.

I used to work in the NHS weight-management service, giving therapy to people before they had weight-loss surgery, and something interesting would often happen after surgery. Many patients were using food to cope – which I would call a food addiction, though some may disagree – but the gastric bypass surgery rendered those patients unable to eat enough to soothe. Their food addiction, in a sense, was cured; however, the pain they were using the food to cope with was not. What we saw was something called 'addiction transference', when one addiction transfers to another. The patients would adopt new addictive coping mechanisms, like alcoholism or gambling. Through this process they found a quick fix for the food issue (the tip of the iceberg), but ultimately the issue was never the food; it was the hole they were trying to fill (the bulk of the iceberg).

So rather than beating yourself up for succumbing to whatever you may be addicted to, try to recognise that your addiction is serving a purpose. It is helping you to cope with something that feels unbearable. The task is to try to connect with what that might be, so you don't need to rely on the addiction any more.

I know this is really hard. It might sound incredibly scary. It did for me too. Unfortunately, sometimes things get a little worse before they get better. That's because to really heal you have to go through all the painful things you have been avoiding.

The antidote to addiction is connection

The opposite of addiction is connection. Connection to other people, and connection to the vulnerable parts of yourself that the addiction is masking. The dopamine and endorphins that we seek through the addiction replace the love and connection we're missing. Addiction fills the void of connection and love. Even if you're surrounded by people, you might not feel deeply connected and loved if you're keeping your more vulnerable parts inside.

The more vulnerable you are with safe people (i.e. the people who can bear and hold your vulnerability), the more connected you will feel. This is what happens in therapy: slowly people start to rely on their therapist and show their pain underneath. The therapist, unlike their parents, does not judge or reject them; they support and accept them. *This is what heals.* We cannot heal alone; healing happens in relationships. This can be done outside of the therapy room, by sharing your feelings with people and allowing yourself to depend on and be depended on by others. The more genuinely connected we feel, and the more community we have around us, the less we need to soothe ourselves with the addiction.

This starts with connecting to yourself.

Just knowing is not enough

Knowing what trauma triggered your addiction is very different from processing the trauma. People tell me all the time, 'I know exactly what my trauma is, but it doesn't help!' They're right, because there's knowing on an intellectual level (e.g. 'I know my abusive father had negative effects on me') and knowing on an emotional level (e.g. feeling how scary it was to have a father who was aggressive and didn't feel safe).

Lana knew what had happened to her, but until she was able to let herself express the confusion she experienced, the disgust and grief and horror, she needed to use work to cope. The same was true for Nathan; he'd always known that the bullying was what led him to start drinking. The work for him was to connect to the feelings of inferiority, isolation and exclusion; the shame he experienced as a young person, which led him to believe there was something wrong with him.

When Nathan first started to talk about his past, he described what happened to him in detail. How he had to partner with the teacher in lessons because no one would dare go near him. The silence that fell when he tried to talk to anyone. Being iced out by the people he thought of as friends. The shame and confusion of the silence. The feeling of being so dirty and repulsive that no one would touch him. It was agonising to listen to. I looked at him, expecting for him to be experiencing the same kind of sadness and discomfort I was feeling, and instead he was beaming at me, sunny and upright, as if he had just told me a story about a cute dog he'd seen. He was not connected to the feeling of the words he'd just told me. Inside, I was feeling it for him.

One of the ways we survive the painful things that have happened to us is by splitting off from all the hurt so we don't have to actually experience it. Entire memories of huge events get pushed down. The number of people who cannot remember large chunks of their childhood is astounding. This stops us from having to face any of the bad things that happened to us. Except they do not go away; they lead us to seek out coping mechanisms even if we can't remember what it is we're trying to cope with.

Healing is the work of rejoining all those separate parts so you can feel whole again, so you don't need the addiction to manage those unwanted parts. The story of what happened is connected to the pain once again. It's hard work to have to feel the things you don't really want to feel. That's why it takes time, repetition and safety.

Things changed for Nathan when he went into work one Thursday and opened his drawer to find that someone had individually wrapped all of his items in wrapping paper. While his office mates sniggered and whispered, Nathan's eyes became thick with tears. He ran to the bathroom to hide his dismay and wept in the cubicle with abandon. His colleagues were alarmed – it was only meant to be a harmless joke, and Nathan was usually light-hearted and playful; they thought he'd take it well. As he tells me what happened, his colleagues laughing as he unwrapped his notebook and pencil, he struggles to get the words out, as if something has its hands around his throat. His jaw tremors, making his speech shaky and almost incoherent. It was seemingly harmless, but Nathan's reaction was disproportionate.

While it might seem as though these feelings are about what's going on in Nathan's present, it feels to me like he's starting to process the past. I cannot tell you how common this is during the healing process. As we start to talk about the bullying he went through, the feelings come to the surface, triggered by the event that mirrored the past. While his colleagues' prank seemed harmless and playful, Nathan is reacting to the bullying from when he was a kid. This is all part of what I understand as 'processing'. While going through the therapy process, you might find yourself getting angry at a partner, when really you're angry at a parent. Or maybe you find yourself crying at a cute child in an advert, when really you might be crying for your own child self.

As we start to put words to the things that have happened to us, it's normal for difficult feelings to come up. By feeling all those vulnerable emotions, we're releasing the stories and shame that have been hiding inside us.

Nathan's desire to drink has not gone away. He still gets triggered, still has cravings to numb himself when he gets overwhelmed. The difference is that Nathan is able to respond differently to those urges. He knows that the impulse to drink is a sign of distress, a sign that he needs to go inwards and connect to the part of him that is crying out to be soothed. 'God, I really want a drink,' he tells me one session after a fight with his partner, Adam. I say nothing, waiting to see how he will make sense of this – the aim as a therapist is not to intervene, not to tell him what to do or what this means, but to help him get there by himself. He looks at me, expectant, waiting for me to scold him or tell him not to. Then he smiles. 'I know what you're going to say: I want the drink to soothe me. I should sit with the feelings, blah blah blah.' I continue to say nothing. 'I guess I'm feeling rejected. Fighting with Adam makes me shut down, like I need to run to protect myself, but drink isn't going to protect me, not really.' I nod, impressed with how far he's come, and feeling somewhat redundant. 'It's funny – if you resist the urge to drink long enough, it turns into something else.'

'What does it turn into?' I ask, intrigued.

'Pain, fear, vulnerability. It's just a little kid, little Nathan, wanting some love. But then, if you stay with that long enough, let the kid have its tantrum, it becomes something quite soft, like relief almost. This whole time I was drinking I was stopping that process, keeping myself from the pain, but also keeping myself from the relief.'

Pride and reverie fill my chest. I have the urge to hug him, or clap (I don't, of course). They tell you when you train to be a therapist that you're not supposed to be too pleased with your patients, because it puts pressure on them to feel they have to be doing well. But sometimes rules are for breaking. Sometimes you have to allow yourself to be moved by people and show them that they have the capacity to move you. So today I let a wide smile fill my face, knowing full well that he might not be 'cured', that he might not always be able to face the pain and find that relief waiting on the other side, that he might drink again one day and have to learn these lessons all over again. He grins back at me, pleased with himself. We sit like this for a while, in silent celebration, nothing more to say.

Tips for connecting to difficult emotions

- **Give yourself permission to feel anything.** Don't try to force how you're feeling. You might feel nothing or feel numb or flat. Maybe you genuinely only feel happy and positive feelings.

- **Tune in to your body.** Feelings are just physical sensations, remember? So, to tune in to your feeling is to tune in to your body. You can do this for yourself. How does your body feel right now? Give yourself a second to check in with yourself. Your body will tell you how it feels, you just need to give it the space.

- **Journal.** Giving yourself a space to write freely whatever you're thinking and feeling can help release emotions you didn't even know you had. Give yourself a few minutes each day just to write, without trying to make it good or imagining that anyone would read it. You're trying to create a place free from judgement where your unconscious is safe to spill out.

- **Connect to your inner child.** Sometimes it's easier to feel empathy for a child than for ourselves. Visualise yourself as a child and try to imagine how they might have felt. Did they always feel cared for? Did they sometimes feel lonely or misunderstood? Try to imagine exactly how it felt for them during the more difficult times. What did that little child need back then? What do they need from you now? The more we visualise and connect to our child selves, the more we can have compassion and empathy for ourselves, and start to connect to that little child's painful feelings, which we might have shut ourselves off from.

SELF-CRITICISM

Why Am I So Hard on Myself?

Why are you such an idiot? Everyone hates you – they're all talking about you behind your back. They think you're annoying, stupid, uninteresting, fat, ugly, irrelevant. Even if you try your best, it will never be good enough. People don't love you, and why should they? You're awful. You're pathetic, too sensitive, too much. You're stupid. It doesn't matter how many achievements you get, whether you do well or not – behind it all you're nothing.

It was uncomfortable to write that, to see those words written down. These are all things I've said to myself. I'm sure you recognise yourself in some of them. The number of people I see who talk to themselves like this on a daily basis, possibly saying even worse things, is heartbreaking.

The strange thing is that none of us would dream of saying such horrible things to other people. I used to run group therapy sessions and we'd do an exercise that deeply affected me every time. Everyone would write out all the worst things they say to themselves on a piece of paper. Then people would get into pairs and say those things out loud to each other, as if saying them about their partner.

In fact, I want you to do the same thing now. Think of the three worst things you say to yourself and say them out loud as if you were saying them to someone else. If you don't have someone near you, imagine saying them to someone instead. Worse, imagine saying them to a little child.

Every time I did this exercise in the groups, they couldn't physically bring themselves to do it, to tell their neighbour they are ugly or boring. It was horrendously uncomfortable to look someone in the eye and tell them they're a horrible, worthless person that no one will ever love. People would often cry, disbelieving that they so freely tell themselves these things that they wouldn't dare say to someone else.

The funny thing is that people in those groups were often in carer roles. They would spend their days as nurses, therapists, teachers, mothers, fathers – easily showing kindness and consideration to others, but completely unable to extend the same compassion to themselves.

Why are we so horrible to ourselves, and so nice to other people? Why could I happily support this group of people, then go home and struggle to do the same for myself?

Why do we have a critical inner voice?

An inner critic is always an outer critic who has been internalised. If you think back to those horrible things you tell yourself, you almost always would have been told them by someone else. We learn what's acceptable and what's not from the people and structures around us.

There are a few different ways we can receive the message that there is something wrong with us:

1. **Directly:** from critical parents, siblings or teachers who tell us off for acting a certain way, make fun of

the things we say or show an interest in, put pressure on us to be successful, pile the expectations on us or criticise what we do.

2. **Through actions:** sometimes the criticisms we absorb are not taught to us through words. Because children are very sensitive to whether they are getting enough care and attention, if they aren't, the child may assume that this is because there's something wrong with them. Maybe Mum was loving and tender with Dad but harsh and dismissive with us. Maybe we saw teachers in school picking on us and not others, or friendship groups excluded us and made us feel inferior. These situations all give us the message that we are not good enough, that we are not as lovable as others.

3. **Indirectly:** maybe the judgements weren't even directed at us. Maybe we overheard Dad making rude comments about people who are stupid and don't have good jobs, making us think he'd be angry if we did badly in school, or maybe Mum would make comments about people's weight, causing us to be harsh on our own bodies when we gained weight.

4. **From society:** even if we have the most loving, supporting parents, we may still learn to criticise ourselves from the conflicting ideas we're receiving from the world about how we should be. We've all been taught that it's better to be thin than fat, nice rather than angry, that women should be feminine and sweet while men should be masculine and unemotional. The list of

messages we receive about the 'right' way to be leave us all inevitably feeling that there is something inherently wrong with us. The message is undoubtably clear: we are not OK as we are.

And what do we do if we're told we are wrong? We try everything we can to be right. We try extra hard in school or do things to impress the cool kids, we fight for attention with our sibling or try our best not to be too much or too needy, or we grow demanding and controlling to try to get our needs met. All the while we're telling ourselves that something is wrong with us, that we're being treated this way because we are deficient.

So, your critical inner voice is weirdly helping you. It's trying to suppress all the parts of you that are considered socially unacceptable. It is the voice of the scared, defended part of you. This means that battling it won't help. Instead of being hard on yourself for being hard on yourself, try to have compassion for that scared part of you that just wants to be liked. The key to quieting it is to introduce a kinder voice that is accepting and compassionate, that eventually drowns out the more critical one.

Fiona

It's clear from our first session that Fiona is furious with herself.

She's a well-put-together woman, grey hair pulled into a neat bun, pressed white shirt and floral skirt. She takes off her blazer, folds it over the chair, then arranges herself in the chair as if she's posing for a photograph. She is meticulous and perfect. I feel self-consciously scruffy in comparison, yet internally, Fiona sees only mess.

Within ten minutes she tells me she hates her ageing body, that she's not good enough for the job she's in, she's too fat, she's a terrible mother and no one will ever love her again. I ask her where she learnt to talk to herself like that, and she stares back as if I've asked her a complex maths problem. 'Learn? I didn't learn it; it's just always been there.'

'What were your parents like?' I ask.

'I'm fifty-nine,' she tells me. 'My parents have nothing to do with this.' In some senses she's right – while the past impacts how we come to be, we don't want to get stuck in the past. Fiona is clearly dealing with pressing issues related to her present and future too.

One of the other things we have to reckon with is the future that lies ahead of us. Time brings change, whether we like it or not. Accepting our own mortality is a challenge for all of us; there is no escaping it. As we age, we all have to wrestle with new identities and loss – of people we love and of the expectations we might have had of our lives.

As her sixtieth birthday approaches, Fiona realises she expected her life to look a lot different to how it is. Having sacrificed her career to raise her kids, she works in a stuffy office with bosses who are half her age. She split from her husband when the kids went to university, and now both her sons live in different countries, leaving her miserable and lonely. She kept waiting for her life to take the form she imagined when she was younger, but it never did. Now, as time trundles on, she is riddled with self-blame and loathing about the failure of her life.

Still, there is something childlike about Fiona that makes me think there is still a young part of her that has got stuck somewhere. It's rare, I find, that people are this self-critical without there being something in their childhood to explain why. Children aren't born criticising themselves; they learn it. There's something fragile about her. I get the feeling that she might break if I push her too hard, so I leave it for now and let her go back to telling me all the ways in which she's failed as a human.

She comes in for her next session red, spluttery and close to tears. Her overly controlling boss has sent her a passive-aggressive email and asked her to come in for a meeting and Fiona is convinced she's going to fire her. She takes a tissue and neatly folds it into a perfect tiny triangle as she talks. While that may be a possibility, there doesn't seem to be much evidence that she's going to be fired, yet Fiona is caught in a swirl of catastrophising. She made a mistake with the accounts, some confidential information got leaked, her latest report wasn't good enough – whatever it is, Fiona is an idiot and is going to suffer the consequences. 'Is there a chance,' I say, 'that you haven't messed up? That this is just an ordinary meeting?'

'No,' she says, squeezing the tissue triangle between her fingers. 'I'm a failure.'

It's sad and difficult to listen to someone berate themselves like this. She tells me she's fat and ugly in nearly every session. Sometimes it's easier for people to express their vulnerabilities in terms of their bodies. It's perfectly acceptable to tell someone you feel fat, and less acceptable to say that you feel horrifically sad or furious or jealous. So all our difficult feelings get put into our bodies, where they can be expressed in a more palatable form.

The same is often true of hypochondria or physical health. We put all our fragility into our bodies, making it feel like they are the problem. If we could just lose weight, look different, get healthy, all our problems would vanish.

This means the source of change is about starting to connect to the things we're using our bodies to express. Underneath 'feeling fat' is usually something more complicated that we aren't able to communicate.

Things to say instead of 'I'm feeling fat'

- I don't feel good about myself.
- I'm feeling like others won't like me as I am.
- I feel sad.
- I'm scared others will reject me.
- I'm feeling pressurised to be a certain way.
- I'm feeling like I'm not enough, not worthy, not lovable.

I want to jump in and tell Fiona that she's beautiful, that she seems caring and funny and smart, but I know that's not my job. My job is to stay with the critical voice and help her get to what's underneath it.

'It seems as though you live in a perpetual state of thinking you're going to get into trouble, and then emotionally beating yourself up,' I say. 'I wonder what it would be like to try to be kind to yourself?'

She snaps. 'Can you stop being so nice to me?' She tears the triangle in two.

'What is it that's so painful,' I ask, 'about me being nice?'

She replies without pause, as if the words have been just on the edge of her lips the whole time. 'I don't deserve it.'

Fiona's ex-husband was often quite cruel to her, humiliating her for her weight and constantly making jibes in front of their friends and kids. Her boss, too, is critical and micromanages everything she does. Even her friends make nasty jokes at her expense and often exclude her from their plans. And Fiona just takes it all, like the punch bag she feels herself to be. It's no coincidence that she ends up in these relationships – she's far more comfortable with being hurt than being loved.

Fiona uses most of the therapy time to attack herself. It's like watching someone repeatedly smack themselves in the face. I try everything. I point out how harsh she is, try to make links to where the voice comes from, offer compassion and empathy, but all my attempts at acceptance and love are rebuffed.

We talk about how she can stand up to some of the people in her life, let them know they're hurting her, set boundaries around the kind of treatment she is and isn't willing to put up with, but nothing changes because ultimately Fiona believes this is the kind of treatment she deserves.

'Are you angry,' I ask, 'that everyone's treating you this way?'

'No,' she says, 'I don't really do anger.'

'Well, you do,' I reply quickly. 'You just only do anger at yourself.' She meets my eye. We share a coy smile. Something has landed.

Body Image

While the culture around our bodies has created a body image crisis, I also think our relationship with our bodies reflects our relationship with ourselves. Caring about how we look is really about how we think others will perceive us and how sensitive we are to rejection. Imagine living in a world with no one else: would you really care about getting wrinkles or having flabby thighs or a big nose? Probably not. A lot of our fears about how we look are actually fears about whether people will accept or like us. Adhering to beauty norms is really about trying to belong. This means that people who haven't always been made to feel loved or accepted will probably be more critical about their bodies.

Fear of rejection can manifest in body image issues because there are such clear societal rules. We're less likely to be rejected if we're pretty and skinny, right? We mostly fear the things that have already happened, so criticising how you look is our mind's way of trying to prevent that initial rejection (probably in childhood) happening again.

The real story emerges later, as Fiona starts to get more comfortable. When Fiona was seven, her mum was sick. She was in and out of hospital and would spend weeks at a time without seeing Fiona. It was terrifying to be without her mum, and Fiona longed for her to return. With her dad often working, Fiona's grandma would come and watch her. Grandma was a stern and religious woman, who carried lots of shame and judgement about how a person, especially a woman, should be. While her grandma didn't directly criticise her, she made it quite clear that there was a certain way to be, and Fiona was not it. All the shame carried by her grandma was poured into her. She was too messy and too loud and not well behaved enough.

Fiona tried everything she could to be good, hoping that if she lived by all of Grandma's rules, maybe her mum would come home. She tried praying, writing letters to the doctors and practising nightly rituals where she'd cast spells to make her mum come home. Sometimes, in her child mind, she wondered if her mum had gone because of her.

Fiona hasn't talked about any of this in years. It's strange to remember the logic of her younger self. She feels cold when she thinks about her grandma, remembering the sinking feeling in her stomach when she would see her floral bag in the hall and smell the lemon-drop scent of the sour lady, knowing that her lovely mum wasn't going to be around for a while. She'd have a flash of anger at her mum – where was she? Why couldn't she just be well like the other mums? But it was too scary to feel mad when her mum was so fragile and her grandma so stern.

When we see our parents as fragile, we don't feel they can bear all our difficult feelings. Children can feel the need to protect their parents, so they keep all these things in. Fiona couldn't tell her mum she was angry that she went away, that she didn't want to be with her grandma or that she was miserable and alone, because she didn't want to overload her mum with more things to worry about.

Instead, Fiona turned all these feelings inwards. She was the problem; it was her fault. Children can sometimes believe they're more powerful than they are. Maybe Fiona believed on some level that she had made her mum ill, or that her mum was staying in hospital because Fiona was too much. And because Fiona felt guilty and afraid of these feelings (what if they made her mum even sicker?), she had nowhere to put them, so they stayed inside. Now, as an adult, Fiona still believes, somewhere deep down, that she is not enough.

Why do kids blame themselves?

I'm going to introduce you to what I think is one of the most important concepts in psychology. It is the thing that makes it so hard to think of our childhoods as anything less than perfect, and also the thing that makes so many of us deeply critical of ourselves. It is called 'the moral defence', first explained by psychiatrist Ronald Fairbairn in 1943[11]. Children who are hurt by their parents will usually blame themselves. This is actually a very clever survival adaptation that keeps the bond with our parents strong. Because we need them to keep us alive, our mind doesn't want to think of them as being bad. This means that when we are treated badly, we assume it's our fault, that we are bad, because thinking of our parents as bad is far too frightening for our survival. We need them to be good in order to feel safe.

Instead, we make it a story about ourselves, rather than them. This way we keep the illusion that we're in control and we believe that if we behave better next time we'll be loved. That means all our anger and hurt gets turned on ourselves. We think we aren't good enough and we become very critical of ourselves. As adults we might think that we're stupid, that no one likes us or we're always feeling guilty about something.

This all happens outside of our awareness – you won't know that you're doing it, but often our critical inner voice comes from this unconscious belief that we are bad, so that we can maintain the belief that our parents are good.

We carry the idea that we are bad into our adult life, and it underpins much of our capacity to love ourselves. We don't feel capable in our studies or at work and put huge pressure on ourselves to do well. We imagine that our friends hate us or our partner secretly thinks we're ugly. We might always think that people are angry at us or that we're going to get into trouble at work, or maybe we tug at our bodies, hating how we look. We're waiting for everyone else to realise the thing we are sure is true: that we are awful people.

Reassurance from others does not help. Even positive affirmations don't really change the way we feel about ourselves, because the feelings are not about us – they are about the caregivers who hurt us. We need to find a way to feel those feelings towards the people who hurt us, so we don't turn that anger and hatred in on ourselves.

The solution is to turn those feelings back onto the people they belong to, the ones who hurt us. It is uncomfortable, but we need to shift the narrative from 'I am bad' to 'I was treated badly', and start to get angry and upset with the people who did that to us.

This is why psychotherapists always harp on about your parents, because they're trying to get you to connect to how let down you may have been by them so you can start to free yourself from blame.

This is also one of the hardest parts of healing. It can feel disloyal to get angry with our parents or see them as bad in any way. However, by refusing to see any flaws, you can end up turning all the anger and blame onto yourself.

Feeling let down doesn't equal blame. It's not Mum's fault she was an alcoholic who shouted; she was shouted at when she was younger. It wasn't Dad's fault he was depressed; his own dad died when he was little. Your parents were once children too, and their mistakes will have a root just like yours.

Just because you're seeing them as flawed, it doesn't mean you don't love them; it just means you're no longer protecting them. We are allowed to feel more than one feeling at once. It can feel really confusing to go through this, but it's a sign of great emotional maturity to be able to feel both love and hate for someone, both pride and envy, both anger and warmth.

If you're reading this and wrestling with these things, I see you. This was, and still is, one of the hardest parts of therapy for me.

It's also been one of the most healing. As I began to realise that there was never anything wrong with me, I was able to stop being so harsh on myself. For many (myself included), once they let themselves feel the full extent of their hurt feelings towards their families, they become more compassionate to their child selves and start to realise that they are not bad at all; they were only made to feel like they were, by people who were probably also once made to feel bad about themselves.

– EXERCISE –

GET CURIOUS: What are the main things you think other people will judge or criticise you for? What are the things your critical inner voice is extra hard on you about?

UNDERSTAND: Where do you think you learnt to talk to yourself like that? Knowing that you're only criticising yourself in ways you've been criticised before (directly or indirectly), try to figure out where you learnt to talk to yourself like this. Can you think of a specific time you felt criticised as a kid, whether directly or indirectly, by your parents, friends, the media, etc.?

FEEL: Your critical inner voice is trying to protect you, remember. Rather than getting angry with yourself for being harsh, try to connect with it. Why do you think it's scared? What are some reassuring things you can tell it (e.g. 'Thanks for trying to protect me, but we don't need to be scared of being too needy, stupid, ugly [insert critical thing here]')?

Why validation doesn't always help

While validation from others can feel good in the moment, it doesn't truly solve the deeper issue. Low self-esteem comes from a wound of not feeling good enough. People can shower you with all the praise and compliments in the world, but it goes through you like a sieve because you don't really believe it to be true. No external validation will ever be enough if you don't love yourself.

That's why external validation from others, though temporarily nice, doesn't solve our self-esteem issues. The problem is coming from the inside.

For some people, validation from others can actually make things worse because there's nothing to project all their negative feelings onto, which can feel very destabilising. In a sense they need a place for their anger and badness to be projected onto (themselves), so when someone compliments them or boosts them up it feels uncomfortable because they need to see themselves as bad in order to believe other people are good.

How can I be less harsh on myself?

As Fiona struggles so much to talk kindly to herself, we introduce Little Fiona into the picture. We start by picturing Little Fiona in the room with us, how old she is, what she's thinking, what she's feeling. Every time Fiona comes to the session with a new round of punches to throw at herself for having been told off by her boss or having gained a few pounds, I remind her of Little Fiona. What's she feeling right now? What would you tell her in this situation?

Her answer is always the same: it's not Little Fiona's fault, she's just a child, she hasn't done anything wrong.

As the blame shifts from her, she starts to have a newfound defensiveness of that little girl. She didn't deserve to be picked on for no reason – she was just a girl. Together we cry for Little Fiona, who was taught she was bad just for existing. She gets angry on Little Fiona's behalf. She wants to go back and defend that little girl, shout at her grandma that she's a bully and rescue her child self. She cannot, of course, but what she does do is take that new-found compassion and start applying it to herself.

Some people call this 'reparenting', which is about connecting to your child self and giving yourself what you needed back then but didn't get. Now, it's important to have compassion for your parents too; they were once children, after all, and being stuck in anger and blame at them isn't helpful either. But by recognising that the things that have happened to you are not your fault, you can release all the hurt you've been taking out on yourself, just like Fiona.

One morning, Fiona bounds into the room and sits in the chair with a fizzing energy I've not seen from her before. 'I did it.' She blows her nose in a tissue, scrunches it carelessly into a ball and tosses it into the bin. 'I was actually nice to myself.'

Her boss sent her yet another belittling email about not doing a task properly and the familiar onslaught began. She was stupid, she wasn't good enough to do this job, she should leave and they'd be better off for it. Then she stopped and remembered Little Fiona. That frightened child inside her who needed love, not hatred. 'We're OK,' she told both her child and adult self, 'we've made a small mistake; it doesn't mean we're bad or stupid.' She sent a confident reply, rather than the usual apology-ridden response, and treated herself to a piece of cake on the way home.

What Actually is Self-love?

I'm not a huge fan of the phrase 'love yourself'; I find it patronising and insincere. That being said, a lot of us do not love ourselves. We say we do: we can tell ourselves positive affirmations, write three things we like about ourselves every day, try to treat ourselves with better self-care. But this is only loving part of ourselves. True self-love is loving the messy bits. It's loving your tendency to be a bit selfish, the envy you feel for your best friend, the bitter or aggressive parts. Self-love is meaningless if you only love the 'good' parts. For true self-love, you have to love the parts you are denying and projecting onto others.

Can you love the parts of you that society, and maybe your family, told you make you unlovable? That's the real test. Can you love the really vulnerable part of you? Can you love the part that sometimes hurts others? If you can start to own and even have compassion for these parts, then you're on the path to real self-love.

Tips to be less harsh on yourself

1. **Try to identify where that critical inner voice comes from.** Who does it belong to? In what way were you made to feel inferior or wrong?

2. **Understand that it was not your fault, that you were made to feel this way.** Being criticised or not accepted as a child is not your problem, but the problem of those who couldn't tolerate themselves.

3. **Connect to the pain of that little child who was made to feel less than good enough.** Hold them in mind when those hateful thoughts appear in your head. Does that little child really deserve to be spoken to in that way? How does it feel for them? Equally, feel what it's like to be the angry, critical part. Might your anger at yourself actually be anger with the people who hurt you? Your anger is justified; it's OK to feel it.

4. **Take active steps to be more compassionate.** When you notice that angry voice, try to counteract it with curiosity rather than believing it. Add in another, more loving and understanding voice to try to counteract the harsh one.

5. **Keep repeating these steps.** The voice will come back – it takes time to be kinder to yourself. The best thing you can do is to keep going through these steps again and again and, over time, the critical inner voice will get a little quieter and the compassionate one will get a little louder.

Part Two:

RELATIONSHIPS

Understanding Relationships

When I was a teenager and first navigating romantic relationships, I thought that love was simple. To me, the hard part seemed to be finding someone in the first place. I imagined that once you'd done the hard work of making yourself look nice, going to the right parties, flirting with someone, telling your friend to ask their friend if they fancy you, crafting the perfect texts to lure them into believing you're cool and chilled, psyching yourself up for a date, trying to show how interesting and cool you are while hiding all the embarrassing parts of yourself and attempting to maintain that new personality you've created each time you see them, the rest of the relationship was easy, right?

As I began studying psychology, with a string of failed relationships under my belt, I came to learn that the movies were wrong: the hard part starts after the first kiss, after the rose-tinted glasses come off and the honey-coated naivety of the honeymoon phase ends. I remember once saying to a partner in the early days, 'There is honestly nothing I would change about you,' only to find myself, after a few years, desperate to change most things about them because we were entirely incompatible and most of their behaviours triggered me.

Relationships are complex, and many of us enter them thoroughly unequipped for the challenges that are about to ensue.

So why are relationships so difficult? Shouldn't it be simple to love someone and stay happy together?

Relationships hold up a mirror to what needs healing. Because romantic relationships are so intimate, they're more likely to mimic family relationships and bring up all the difficulties we've faced in our childhood. It is in our romantic relationships that we have to face conflict, difficult conversations, struggles with vulnerability, issues around boundaries, sex and compromise. They trigger us and open us up. Relationships force us to face ourselves.

This is a blessing and a curse. It makes relationships a potential source of pain, but also a source of immense growth. If you can reflect on your relationships, you can learn more about yourself. Many of us heal through relationships, by becoming more aware of how we show up for other people, reflecting on what we can do differently and then trying to choose new ways of being.

The world would be a far kinder and easier place if we were all taught at school the fundamentals of how to be in a healthy relationship. We learn how to be in healthy relationships by doing. Then messing up, learning and trying again. When we lack fundamental knowledge about ourselves, and how relationships work, we end up projecting our unwanted parts onto other people, chasing people who aren't good for us or choosing people who repeat our childhood wounds. The way we learn about ourselves is by experiencing ourselves in relation to another. This means that relationships will always be a big part of the growing process. We just need to make sure we stay curious and try to learn from our experiences by taking accountability for our part, rather than shaming ourselves or the other person for what went wrong.

My teenage self found relationships difficult because she'd never done them before. And, probably, if I hadn't had years of therapy and reflection, I'd be making the same mistakes that she did. That's not to say that I'm now an exemplary participant in my relationships; I'm still learning, as we all are. But what I do know is that good relationships take dedication and practise. We should be constantly reflecting on what goes well and what doesn't, and becoming more aware of our patterns and our past, so that we can learn from what hasn't gone well and strive to do things differently next time.

We will never be perfect – messing up is inevitable – but at least we can try to make relationships a little easier for ourselves.

Now, if you're anything like me, you're going to read this next part of the book with a certain someone in mind. You're going to think about everything that's wrong with them and everything you can do to change them. Be honest with yourself: how many times have you thought, 'If they would just change this one thing, everything would be great'?

Focusing on changing another person is ultimately a way to avoid ourselves. What you may not realise is that while you're googling how to make someone commit or be less avoidantly attached or stop being so narcissistic, change in your relationship is becoming far less likely, because the only thing we can change is ourselves.

We have to understand this. Sometimes it means walking away from a situation that isn't working, sometimes it means taking accountability for our side of things, sometimes it means raising difficult conversations or setting boundaries. I'll go through all of these things in this section, but I implore you to do what it took me years to figure out: as you read through the following pages, focus on yourself. Don't use this information to try to fix the person you are dating as you will be wasting your time. Reflect on *your* feelings, *your* patterns, *your* behaviours. This introspection is what creates change.

In dating, you can't really get things 'wrong' or 'right', you can only learn. And you learn by having relationships and new experiences of being with different types of people and assessing what feels good to you. Rather than seeing every situation as a problem or minefield, try to see every new connection and first date as an opportunity to get to know yourself better. It's all an experiment for you to learn what you like, what you don't like, what your patterns are, what triggers you and, ultimately, who you are.

That being said, dating makes us feel very vulnerable. It evokes our primal needs and fears – wanting to be loved, the fear of being rejected, the risk of being hurt, the fear of ending up alone. So, while in theory it's all a learning experience, it's also normal to feel triggered and challenged. Be gentle with yourself and try to stay curious – and maybe even enjoy yourself along the way.

Of course, *all* relationships have their challenges, but for this section I'm going to focus mainly on romantic relationships, because they tend to be the place where we struggle the most.

I'm going to go through some of the most common relationships issues and patterns I see. This list is not exhaustive – there are countless ways relationships can give us grief – but I will try to cover some of the core issues, what could be underneath them and what might help.

Section One
Being Single

GOING SOLO

How Can I Be Happy on My Own?

I get asked this question frequently, and it's one I have struggled with myself in the past. We are a relationship-driven species; this means we are wired for love. In our modern society most of us no longer live in communities, which creates a pretty lonely way of life. We live in separate houses, eat lunch at our desks, call our parents every couple of weeks, meet friends for rushed drinks and then go back home alone again. It is no surprise so many of us are focused on romantic relationships to fulfil our need for connection.

On top of all this isolation, we are then told to be happy on our own and not obsess over being in a relationship. How do we meet our need for closeness and intimacy while also being strong and independent? Denying our natural need for a relationship should not be a point of pride. We all need people; we all need relationships to survive. Let's not shame ourselves by thinking we're needy or desperate for wanting a relationship. Needing relationships is just as valid as needing to eat or breathe.

If you're single and trying to suppress your need for connection, you will likely experience loneliness and then shame for feeling lonely. I always think about my dog when I think about loneliness. We all know it's cruel to leave a dog on their own. They're pack animals and most people say, 'You shouldn't leave them for more than a few hours, or they'll get sad.' So, what about humans?! Humans are more social than dogs, and yet no one thinks it's cruel to leave us on our own for more than a few hours. Of course, being alone is normal and can be very nourishing, but why are we constantly encouraged to be happy on our own? We are not made to be completely independent from each other; we're made for connection.

A list of things I've told myself when I've been single:

- I'm desperate.
- I should be happy on my own.
- I'm of no value unless I'm in a relationship.
- Everyone feels sorry for me.
- Clearly no one will ever love me.
- I don't need anyone.
- I'm too needy.

See how much shame there is? You can't win – either you're wrong for wanting a relationship or wrong for being on your own. And these judgements aren't things I've plucked out of thin air; they're doctrines I've absorbed from the culture around me. From my family setting me up with people who were clearly not right for me, to being excluded from couples-only events, to social media telling me to be strong and independent, the pressure to be both coupled up immediately and simultaneously comfortable in my singledom is painful and confusing. Let me be clear: there is nothing wrong with wanting to be single, and there is nothing wrong with wanting a relationship.

But don't you have to love yourself before you can love somebody else?

People say you need to be happy on your own before you can be in a healthy relationship, but I disagree. I think people can find great healing from within romantic relationships. You don't learn to love yourself by avoiding love. Relationships are where we heal.

I'm not saying you *need* to be in a romantic relationship to heal, or that you can't heal if you're single, but I want to debunk the myth that you have to love yourself before being in a relationship. Growth takes place when we are confronted with the same triggers and deal with them differently. Healing is daring to face those triggers, not avoiding them.

We are relational creatures; we need others to feel safe. This doesn't only mean romantic relationships; growth can happen in any relationship. You learn to love yourself by letting yourself be loved by others. So don't feel like you can't risk love if you're still working on yourself. Love might be the very thing you need.

One of the reasons why being single can be so difficult, and romantic relationships can cause such pain, is because our individualistic society tells us that all of our needs should be met by our romantic partners. This makes it impossible to find someone who ticks every box. We're relying on one person to meet the needs a whole village used to. The expectations we have of our partners to be our best friend, our financial partners, our housemates, our family and our sexual partner is nigh on impossible.

It also means that when we aren't in a relationship, we feel by default that we are missing someone to fill all those roles.

The natural implication of this is that when someone shows us interest we might feel compelled to jump into a relationship with them, just so we don't have to feel the loneliness that comes with being single in our current society.

Build yourself a village

Being happy on your own requires building yourself a village, so you can feel connected outside of a romantic relationship. Lean in to your friendships, take up new interests or nurture old friendships that have fallen by the wayside. Book holidays, visit your family more, reach out when you're feeling lonely. This is the time to consider the quality of the connections we have, not necessarily the frequency. Seek out relationships where you can be vulnerable. Attend sharing circles or groups where you can really be authentic and connect on a deeper level.

Then, down the road, if a romantic interest comes along, you can evaluate whether they are a healthy match for you from a place of fulfilment and abundance, rather than throwing yourself at the first person who shows you interest because you're completely starved of connection. When our needs are met by lots of other people and different areas of our lives, there's less pressure on our romantic lives. We can then choose to stay single or to enter into a new relationship without being driven by desperation for any kind of connection.

– *EXERCISE* –

What are the expectations you have of a potential partner? Write them down here (and be honest):

How can you fulfil some of these needs outside of a romantic relationship? Are there other relationships you can nurture that might help take the pressure off your potential partner?

Think of three things you can do for yourself that create romance, love and connection:

1. ______

2. ______

3. ______

Do I have to be in a relationship to be healthy?

Because our culture is so relationship-obsessed, we might have been made to think that being in a relationship is a necessity for our health and happiness. This is not the case. You might be reading this thinking, 'But I love being single!' There is absolutely nothing wrong with that – there is no shame in wanting to be on your own. Being single doesn't mean you're closing yourself off from love; you can still love and be loved in your relationships. Some people genuinely prefer being on their own, and that is completely valid (you just have to ignore the copious messages from Hollywood, Disney, your parents, your friends, social media, Valentine's Day, and everything else in between).

For some people, romantic relationships are too painful to endure, and they are far more content and balanced being single. If you tend to lose yourself in relationships, being on your own might feel like the only way you can maintain your sense of self and put your own needs first. Ironically, being single is often the most stable I've felt – there's no complicated relationship to play with my emotions and I find it easier to maintain my sense of wholeness when I'm on my own. Relationships are difficult – they trigger you and hold up a mirror to all your patterns. When I've been single (and not pining after someone), I've actually felt more connected to myself than when I've been in the wrong relationship.

That being said, avoidance might not be a long-term solution if a relationship is something you want. Many people are sabotaging relationships because, unconsciously, they're afraid. If you're staying single because you're avoiding intimacy or because relationships are too painful, there may be some unhealed wounds that need attention to make your experience of relationships a little less difficult. While you're working on yourself, you can still find connection and romance in your other relationships. Maybe these can even be a place of healing for you before you brave the intensity of a romantic relationship.

FANTASY RELATIONSHIPS

Sometimes Fantasy is Easier Than Reality

For some, it's safer and more comfortable to stay single and live in fantasy relationships, even if consciously they want to be with someone.

Jay tells me, in no uncertain terms, that he has ruined his own life. He's been desperate to find the one all his life. He finally found her, and then he blew it. That's why he's here – to get her back and to stop it from happening again.

He's been a hopeless romantic since he was young. He was the kid at school picking roses for the girls and proposing in the playground. His older sister used to tease him about always coming home with a different girlfriend, and she never lets him forget the time he accidentally ended up with two dates to the school disco and had to pretend he was sick to stop them finding out. His friends also make fun of him for being so soft and falling in love the moment a girl looks at him.

He knows he falls hard, but he can't get enough of that feeling of being in love. It's been two whole months since his last relationship and he's ready to meet someone. He downloads the apps and starts going on dates, planning salsa evenings and moonlit walks along the canal. The dates are a hit, but the girls are not. There's nothing wrong with any of them per se, but he's looking for the endgame, for fireworks, for that heart-stopping feeling that makes time stand still. It's a numbers game, someone tells him, so he ups the ante and schedules five dates in a week. Still, no one lights him up in the way he wants.

On one of the not-so-great dates at a local jazz bar, a woman wearing a velvet suit and bright orange bra under the blazer gets up on stage. Her name is Yaz, she tells the audience in a husky voice. Elegantly, she glances in his direction with a coy smile, then opens her mouth to sing. Jay is transfixed. The way she moves as she sings, self-assured yet vulnerable. His eyes won't leave her mouth. His date asks a question about where he works, and he blinks himself back into the room, stealing a final glance at Yaz before he answers. He knows nothing about this woman, other than the fact that he needs her.

After he walks his date to the bus stop, he runs back to the jazz bar, praying she's still there. He sees the guitar case propped up on the bar first and grins in celebration. Then he coughs, smooths down his T-shirt and sits down next to her . . .

Their love is everything he's been craving: passionate, sexy, all-encompassing. He cannot get enough. His sister teases him about how fast things are going, but he assures her this is the one. They meet each other's friends; she meets his mum; after a few weeks they even talk about moving in together. Maybe this really is the big love he's been dreaming of. Then Yaz makes a joke about being his wifey. There's a glimmer of irritation in his belly; he ignores it. Then he notices that Yaz has a habit of saying 'that's so funny' instead of laughing. It irritates him slightly, but he ignores that too. In bed, they're arm dancing to an unknown techno track he proudly plays her, then Yaz puts on K-pop. 'You're joking,' he says, more an instruction than a question. She is serious. Can he really be with someone who's into trashy music? The differences only snowball. Yaz said she might want to move to a different country one day; he wants to stay home. Maybe they're not as compatible as he hoped.

He worries to his friends that Yaz might not be quite as great as he once thought, and they tell him he's crazy. 'She's perfect for you. Don't throw away a good thing – again.' But the niggling feeling does not leave. One night he finds himself drunk in a club. A girl is making eyes at him. He knows he shouldn't, but something takes over, a force greater than him, which suspends all the guilt and shame he's going to feel tomorrow morning. He kisses her.

It's only a matter of time before Yaz finds out and breaks up with him, distraught. Except, in the end, it's Jay who is bereft. When Yaz leaves she takes the memories of her flaws with her, leaving behind the idealised version he cannot have. The problems that once plagued him seem irrelevant. What was he thinking? It doesn't matter that she likes different music or has annoying habits. She was his soulmate, everything he'd ever wanted. Why did he mess things up like that?

We can call Jay a narcissist, a cheater, a callous, self-centred idiot. Those things may well be true, but they are the tip of the iceberg. Under the surface, Jay has unconscious motivations for ruining things. He sabotaged this for a reason, he just doesn't know it yet. Why do we do this? Why do we sabotage the things we know are good for us and will make us happy?

What's going on underneath?

This feels to me like a classic case of self-sabotage. As soon as things got real with Yaz, it felt scary for Jay.

Remember, our mind doesn't care about happiness; it only cares about survival. So, if the thing you desire is seen to be threatening, your unconscious will sabotage it for you.

Why would Jay think that being with Yaz is a threat to his survival? Surely being in a happy relationship will benefit him, right? Unfortunately, Jay explains that he didn't have the happiest of experiences in his early relationships. He grew up in a rough area, on an estate rife with violence and crime. He was a smart and happy kid, who formed strong friendships with the boys at school. His best friend, Malik, was his ride or die. Their mums were best friends, too, and the boys grew up together as brothers. As teenagers they'd spend hours laughing together over stupid videos, sit next to each other in every lesson, counsel each other about how to talk to girls. Malik was part of every family photo, every Christmas day, every non-eventful day, every memory and story from his life.

Until they were fourteen, when the worst happened. Malik was in the wrong place at the wrong time. Jay remembers getting the call from his mum. He was trying to pull the knife out of someone's hand, and got caught in the cross-fire.

Malik's death broke Jay. He didn't speak for three months, too afraid to open his mouth in case he shattered from the pain that came out. He didn't say it enough, but Jay had never loved anyone more than he'd loved Malik. That kind of loss can't be repaired, can't ever be replaced. He worked through the grief and moved on – he had to – but his heart never healed, not really.

Now, as an adult, Jay doesn't let himself get close to anyone like that again. Traumatised from the loss, the scared part of him sabotages things when they get serious because it's terribly afraid of being hurt again. Though he craves love and really believes he wants a relationship, he simply can't risk that kind of pain.

Self-sabotage happens when your unconscious and your conscious are in disagreement – when we consciously think we want to do one thing, but our unconscious does the opposite.

You might desperately want a relationship, but if you've learnt as a kid that being close to people is dangerous because they let you down or disappear, your unconscious will sabotage any hopes you have of building happy relationships. If you want to stop smoking or drinking, but your mind has learnt that it's the best way to keep your feelings down, it will make it very hard to stop.

What happened with Jay?

Jay attaches to the therapy almost as quickly as he attached to Yaz. Everything I said was *amazing*, every session was *transformative*. He'd think intensely in between sessions, and come in bursting with new memories and thoughts he'd been storing up to tell me. He oohs and aahs as I speak, eyes wide like a little boy eating ice cream for the first time.

This intensity can happen when someone starts thinking about themselves for the first time; there's a hope and an excitement about seeing things from a whole new perspective and having someone listen to you, often for the first time in your life. But there's something about Jay's obsessive applause that feels a little unreal. Is he idealising me just as he idealised Yaz? I won't lie, being idealised like this is a nice ego stroke, but it's also a lot of pressure, as if everything I say has to be perfectly attuned and insightful so as to live up to his version of me.

Then the inevitable happens: I get something wrong. I call him by the wrong name. It's a slip of the tongue, which I take back and apologise for in a second, but the damage is done. His disappointment is palpable. I can see it in the way his body stiffens, how his eyes fall to the corner of the room, refusing to meet mine. 'I'm sorry,' I say again. 'You seem hurt.'

'It's fine,' he replies, eyes still fixed to the corner. His withdrawal is aggressive; I feel like I've committed a terrible sin, of which there is no possibility of repair.

He doesn't come to the next session. I wonder if he's angry with me, if it's too difficult to come and communicate that to me, if he's punishing me by staying away. Then I get the email: 'Dear Annie, I can no longer come to the sessions, thanks for everything.'

It took me a while to understand what happened, and I might never fully know, but I suspect that, just like Yaz, Jay couldn't tolerate my imperfections.

For some people, especially those who have been let down badly in the past, people are seen as either good or bad. This is the case even if the person didn't intend to hurt you, or leaves through no fault of their own. Malik's death taught Jay that people he loves will leave him, and therefore people cannot be trusted. As soon as someone hurts you (even if unintentionally) or makes a mistake, our child brains assume they are no longer good and can't be trusted. In reality, people are not good or bad; all of us are capable of hurting people and making mistakes, even if we try our best and don't intend to. When we idealise people as Jay did with me and Yaz, we're protecting ourselves from the possibility that they will one day mess up and hurt us. To be in close relationships with people, we have to risk getting hurt.

Though consciously he wanted therapy and was finding it helpful, Jay found the closeness and vulnerability of the relationship too risky. So as soon as I made a mistake and fell down from my pedestal, I imagine it became too frightening for him to stay and risk me hurting him again.

I was left with a feeling of dissatisfaction and sadness that I wasn't able to help Jay with this and talk about how I'd upset him and how we could move through it. Jay's initial idealisation of me was a fantasy. Therapists are never perfect – no one is. If Jay had stayed and learnt to accept that people sometimes get things wrong, and that this is something you have to learn to tolerate if you want to be close to people, then maybe he would have learnt to find a way to move from fantasy relationships to the Big Love he so desperately wanted.

Why do we have fantasy relationships?

Fantasy relationships are a defence against intimacy. While we are living in our heads, we are not risking real love.

Love is terrifying. We're vulnerable when we let ourselves love someone. We're risking them changing their mind, moving away, cheating with someone else, dying. I can't stress enough how many of us are sabotaging romantic relationships because deep down we're so afraid of getting hurt. This is especially true if you've been hurt before, as children or adults. We expect the same will happen again, leaving us reluctant to let someone in.

Chasing someone unavailable, who we've created an entire relationship with in our head, is a way to minimise this risk.

We might say we want a relationship, we might date fanatically and obsess about being with people, but our behaviour tells a different story. We sabotage relationships, choose unavailable people, reject people who like us and chase the ones who don't.

While much of what I've told you so far involves looking backwards to understand ourselves, sometimes our issues aren't just about the past, but about the future and what it holds. The future brings time and getting older and the loss that comes with it. Underneath fantasy relationships can sometimes be a desire to stay as children, connected still to our parents. Many of us don't want to have to grow up and enter into adult relationships with all the intimacy and potential pain they might bring.

Let's break down some of the reasons we run from relationships, by looking at the past, present and future.

1. **PAST.** We've been hurt badly in the past, whether by our parents, friends in school, past relationships. If we've learnt that relationships bring us pain, we will expect every relationship to go the same way. Fantasising about and chasing people we can't have or who don't like us back stops us from having to go through all that pain again.

2. **PRESENT.** We don't want to be in the present. In the present we feel lonely and ashamed that all our friends

are in relationships when we are single. Maybe we don't want to feel that pain, so we create stories where life is different, without shame or loneliness. Or maybe we're in a relationship but stuck in the fantasy that they'll be different; we don't want to accept the present experience of being with that person, because if we did, we'd have to leave. We live in a fantasy to avoid reality.

3. **FUTURE.** We don't want to grow up. If we haven't yet separated emotionally from our parents, it makes it hard to have serious adult relationships. If you were very close to your parents, but they tended not to see you as a separate person, you might still be 'enmeshed' with them. This is usually the kind of relationship that has merged boundaries, where you feel responsible for your parents' feelings and struggle to have different opinions or do things they don't approve of. Often when we're still enmeshed with our parents, it can be challenging to develop adult romantic relationships, because part of us doesn't want to move on from our families.

How to move away from fantasy relationships

To move out of fantasy relationships and into real ones, it's important to recognise that there is a part of you that is probably afraid of being in a real relationship. Identify and name what you're afraid of. Trace back through the relationships that have hurt you and get in touch with the scared, vulnerable part of you. By owning and accepting that part, you're less likely to run. You can then reflect on what your fantasies are showing you – they can teach you what you do want. Reflect on your fantasies, learn what it is that's missing in your life and try to find ways to fulfil those desires, whether that's through romantic relationships or something else.

Then, try to meet those needs through other means. Find a friend to share hobbies or experiences with to gain more security in your sense of who you are; find ways to feel more intimate with yourself or others. If we can meet our needs outside of a relationship, there will be much less pressure on it matching our wild fantasies.

And if a relationship is something you want, you have to take the risk. That means staying even when people aren't perfect, trying your best to make things work, challenging your internal saboteur when it kicks in. Yes, opening yourself up to love means that you might get hurt, but I promise you will be OK, because even if things go wrong, you will have yourself. And there is no one who can take that away from you.

LONELINESS

How Can I Feel Less Lonely?

One of the main reasons people fear being single is loneliness. While that's a very common and understandable worry, being single doesn't necessarily mean you're lonely, and being in a relationship doesn't necessarily mean you aren't. There's nothing lonelier than being in a relationship where you're not connected to someone, where you have to hide parts of yourself or fight for attention. Loneliness is about more than just whether we're in the physical presence of another – it runs a little deeper than that.

The connection we have to ourselves is the best predictor of how deeply we can connect to others. If you want deeper connections with people, start getting to know yourself.

For me, loneliness is about how seen and understood you are. I've had times in my life when I've had a thriving social life, was surrounded by people, yet still felt indescribably lonely because I wasn't being my authentic self, so no one ever really saw the real me. I wasn't doing this consciously – I was barely aware that I wasn't being my authentic self, because I wasn't even showing it to myself. I just felt empty and disconnected.

The cure for loneliness is true connection. This means taking off our mask and being vulnerable. We all want to be seen, but we can only do this if we dare to show ourselves.

Unfortunately, this is easier said than done, because we are wearing those masks for a reason – our unconscious child selves believe they are keeping us safe, because they did back then. But now, as adults, they're keeping us lonely and disconnected.

What does it mean to be your true self?

The idea of a true and false self was first proposed by paediatrician and psychoanalyst Donald Winnicott[12]. The idea is that people form a false self that is a kind of social mask we develop to protect our more vulnerable, real selves. The false self is how we've learnt to adapt to our families and to society. It's when we laugh at a joke that actually hurt us, do things other people want even if we don't want to, stay quiet when we're feeling upset, wear clothes we don't like in order to fit in, smile instead of getting angry.

The more we feel accepted by our parents as kids, the more we'll feel loved and accepted for our true selves. Our parents may not have been perfect, but if we learnt that our most honest needs and feelings were OK, we'll grow up with confidence that we can be our true selves. That if we cry someone will do their best to be there and understand us.

If we don't feel accepted or get enough attention for whatever reason – your parent was ill, depressed, distracted, not around, or maybe you weren't accepted on a societal level for being queer, trans, bigger bodied, from a minority ethnic group, etc. – we'll develop a false self where we behave how we think other people want us to, rather than how we authentically are. This is where people-pleasing can stem from – we think we need to be good and obedient and palatable in order to be loved, so our true self gets pushed down.

I think of this as a scale – how big our false self is compared to our true self. Here are some signs that your false self is strong:

- You feel lonely even when with people.
- You're very aware of people's feelings and how you should act in social situations.
- You don't often have strong emotions, and if you do, you don't show them to others.
- You feel the need to think positively and struggle with negativity.
- You're focused on your image and worry about what people think of you.
- You don't feel present.
- You live a successful life, but inside you feel empty.
- You struggle to be vulnerable.
- You find yourself saying 'I'm fine' a lot.

If these resonate with you, it might be the case that you're wearing a social mask a lot of the time, which can really get in the way of your connection to others and to yourself. Many of us have no idea who we really are – our false selves are so good that we don't even know the difference between what's false and what's real. We then build relationships based on our false selves, but something feels missing or empty.

Loneliness can often be an echo of an earlier experience of having to hide your true self. Your inner child may be remembering a time when they had to hide who they were. Some of us have not taken off our social masks since we were children, so inside sits a very lonely child who is longing to be seen.

Try to connect to that child, to be the one to see them, and then slowly begin to show that child to others. This is the best way to feel connected. Even if it's terrifying and unfamiliar, at least you won't feel as alone.

How to connect to your authentic self

Connecting to your authentic self is about feeling more whole, letting in those vulnerable feelings so you feel more alive. It's about getting in touch with what you really want, rather than what you've been told you want, and then showing up in the world unapologetic for who you really are. To really let go of that mask, we have to learn that it's safe to show ourselves.

I know this is all very easy for me to say, and so much harder and scarier to actually do – believe me, I've been there. But the relief and freedom of meeting your vulnerable self, and then showing that person to others, is truly life-changing.

This is where therapy comes in. Therapy is a safe place where you can practise being your authentic self without the negative consequences you expect (hopefully). It's about learning that it's safe to be real, giving your true self a place to show itself without being judged for being too selfish or angry or bad. It's a place where, sometimes slowly, the walls of the false self can begin to come down so you can meet the more vulnerable person who's been hiding all these years. This will allow you not only to connect more deeply to yourself, but, as you start to show that vulnerability to others, to form stronger connections to other people too.

If therapy isn't an option, try to get those needs met in the present by showing your vulnerability to a safe person and nourishing that part of you that has been in hiding all your life and desperately wants to be seen.

Tips to feel less lonely

1. **Try to connect to what you're hiding.** Are there any dark or deep parts you're ashamed of? Why do you think you can't share those things with other people? Are you afraid those things will make you less lovable or acceptable? The parts you're most ashamed of are the ones that need the most compassion. Try to find a way to accept those parts so they no longer need to hide in the shadows.

2. **Take off your mask.** Tell people how you really feel. The more vulnerable we are, the closer we are to being understood.

3. **Find a community of like-minded people.** Seek out relationships in which you can really be yourself. It's easier to be open and vulnerable with new people, where those old patterns aren't entrenched, so seek out spaces where you might find them.

4. **Help someone.** We all want to feel wanted. By giving to others and experiencing their recognition and gratitude, we often feel more connected.

5. **Try to be more present.** Feeling less lonely is about first connecting to yourself. Whether it's mindfulness, breathwork, physical exercise, journaling, talking to yourself, dancing – try anything that brings you into the present moment.

Section Two
Finding a Relationship

DATING

A High-stakes Game

Meera is a successful person. She's excelling in her career as an interior designer, she's just put down a deposit for a flat that she's going to do up herself, she's got a close-knit friendship group she has stayed close to since university, she might even get a new puppy soon. Despite all this, Meera can't quite figure out her love life.

Meera is a serial dater. Her last relationship was three years ago, and since then she's been in a string of situationships (see page 198) that all seem to meet the same fate. The pattern is indisputable. She goes on a flurry of different dates, hating each one. They're either too dull or too short or talk too much or are obsessed with football. She wants an intelligent man, a creative man, someone she can really connect to.

Then, out of nowhere, one comes along. And she falls hard and fast.

Eddie becomes the most interesting person she's ever met. Within a few dates she's obsessed and is telling all of her friends that she is in love. They roll their eyes – she says this every time. This time, she means it.

And she does. She really does love him. They text all day, his jokes are the funniest she's ever heard, he has the best music taste and the sexiest smile. Even the sex is better than with anyone else. It's wild and passionate and urgent. He's not like the others; he's exciting and present and real.

Then something shifts. She's not sure what – it would be imperceptible to most people, but she can sense something's off immediately. He takes a little longer to reply, makes fewer suggestions to meet up, seems distracted when they're together. The familiar whirring of anxiety kicks in. It must be something she's doing. She tries carefully to seem like she's chilled, but to her friends it's clear she's fallen off the deep end. Screenshots of messages; hours spent crafting perfect replies; deleting his number so she doesn't text him too quickly; overthinking what to wear, what to say, how to be.

She messages more, suggesting ideas for dates and hoping it will keep Eddie interested. He continues to pull away, but it's subtle. So subtle that her friends tell her it's in her head. But she knows rejection when she sees it. If she could just get some security from him, maybe she'd feel better. His replies get shorter and the dates more infrequent.

She becomes deranged, obsessed with luring him back, quite sure that he'll be interested again if he could just remember how good they were together. Except now it's been three weeks since they saw each other, and his 'sorry, been busy' messages are starting to seem insincere. Meera is in agony. She talks of nothing else. Her friends try to be supportive, but she can tell they're sick of this. And so is she. She really thought this time was different, yet here she is again, obsessed with a man who doesn't seem to care. There's no sign of the confident, independent woman she was before they met. She's reduced to a miserable, anxious wreck.

Why does this keep happening to her? Why do these men show interest and then ghost her when she starts to fall for them? Is she giving out the wrong message? Why can she be so successful in the rest of her life, but then completely fail at relationships?

I see many people like Meera, who are doing very well in most areas, yet still struggle in their romantic relationships.

Why are romantic relationships so challenging?

It can be easy to hide our deeper struggles from other people, and from ourselves, but the place they cannot hide is in our relationships. If you are suffering within yourself, your relationships will suffer too.

To be human is to be in relation to one another. None of us exist in a vacuum (as much as some would like to!). That means that any problems going on inside you become problems for your relationships.

I didn't quite understand this until I started working as a therapist and found that relationships were the most common thing that people struggled with (not just romantic, but also family, friends, colleagues). Yes, people have their moods and their addictions, their despair and their anxieties, but all of these play out on the battlefield of relationships, whether it's navigating the impossible world of dating, a difficult friend, a mother who doesn't approve of their choices, a son they can't connect to or a wife who nags them too much. When people come to see me, they bring their relationships with them.

This also means they bring their past relationships. The people who gave them their blueprint for what a relationship is supposed to look like. When they sit in that chair, they sit as their present selves, but also as their baby self, their child self, their teen self. And in the room with us are all the people who shaped them during those years. Their parents, their school peers, their teachers, their siblings, their heroes, their friends, their foes.

And, of course, there is the relationship between the therapist and the patient.

The number one predictor of success in therapy is the strength of the relationship between the therapist and the patient. In a meta-analysis of meta-analyses (basically the crème de la crème of scientific research), a good therapeutic relationship has been shown to lead to far better outcomes in therapy.[13] If this is not proof that relationships are everything, I don't know what is.

Relationships are at the core of healing, but they are also at the core of suffering. Most traumatic things that happen do so within our relationships.

Remember, when we are babies, relationships are the only thing sustaining our life and protecting us from death. A problematic or lacking relationship in those early years can completely terrify and traumatise a child, because it can feel almost deadly.

The trouble with dating

Why is it that romantic relationships are the hardest? Why can Meera have a good relationship with her sister, a whole host of friends who love her and colleagues who respect her, yet she has no success in love?

One reason is because, in adulthood, the stakes are far higher in romantic relationships. The threat of being abandoned or rejected is far bigger in romantic relationships than in any other. We don't enter into friendships with the expectation that we will break up (though friendship break-ups are devastating – more on that later; see page 289). Romantic love is really the only kind of love where we approach it anticipating failure. As a result, our fear responses are exaggerated.

A friend not texting us back might not bother us at all, but a romantic partner taking all day to respond can drive us crazy, because we're more sensitive to rejection from them.

After all, potentially we have to see this person every day, share our finances with them, maybe create a family with them, have them get on with everyone we know, find them attractive, live with them and have good sex with them. All of these demands and expectations make romantic relationships uniquely complicated. Plus, the more intimate our relationships, the more they mirror our family relationships, which bring up a whole host of old patterns and triggers.

SEXUAL CHEMISTRY

Is Intense Chemistry a Good Thing?

Once Meera feels she's ready to move on from Eddie, she tentatively dips her toe in the dating water once again. After a run of mediocre dates with guys she doesn't find interesting, she matches with someone she can already tell is too far out of her league. Meera sees him sitting at the bar with a negroni and nearly turns back out of the door. He's clearly far too cool for her. He shows up with headphones around his neck, a frayed denim jacket and peroxide hair reflecting in the dim light. Meera is wearing a blouse and skinny jeans with her bike helmet dangling from her backpack. This is not going to go well. Her stomach flips as she approaches.

Three drinks in and he's throwing his head back at her lame puns. He brushes his fingers on hers as he reaches for the menu. 'Another drink?' he asks. Meera can't be sure but it seems like he actually likes her. Someone like him wouldn't be interested in someone like her, surely? As he reads the menu she lets her gaze fall on him for a little longer. There's something aloof about him that makes him seem mysterious. He has this kind of nonchalance that makes her wonder if he's interested at all. Then he'll catch her eye or touch her arm and energy will fizz through her. She wants to know everything about him.

As the night closes and they walk to the station, she gives herself a pep talk. 'Kiss him – men like an assertive woman.' Fear coursing through her body, she cups his cheek, eyes locked, and their lips meet. It's the kind of kiss people write songs about, all passion and sex and the merging of souls. Meera can literally feel the sparks fly between them. She smiles coyly and says she'll see him again soon.

'I think I'm in love,' she says to me.

'What's his name?' I ask, realising she hasn't said it.

'Jay.'

I wait until Meera leaves to freak out. Is it the same Jay? The one who idealised people and then ran away when things got too real? They both live near my therapy room, so it's not entirely unrealistic that they would have met somehow. I trawl back through Meera's description – into music, denim jacket, mixture of intensity and aloofness. It all adds up.

My first thought is for Meera: based on what I know about Jay, this is not going to end well. My second thought is for me: is this ethical? What are the rules about patients dating your ex-patients? I book an emergency session with my supervisor to discuss what to do. The general rule is that you shouldn't see patients who have any kind of relationship. Your therapist is supposed to be entirely objective and separate from their life, which enables us to help see situations from a more neutral point of view and maintain perspective. It's also better to keep the boundaries straightforward. Imagine if I was seeing both Meera and Jay; how on earth would I stay objective without getting in the middle of things? On the one hand, it's a small world and these things do happen more than you think. But on the other, Jay is no longer a patient, so it's technically OK. Still, something feels strange about the fact that I've worked with him, that I know all about Yaz and his previous relationships.

I can't tell Meera what I know, because I have to protect confidentiality with Jay. So, my supervisor and I decide not to do anything for now. I'll try to stay neutral when Meera talks about Jay and wait to see how things unfold.

To Meera's surprise, Jay messages to arrange a second date, but she is busy; he's a touring musician doing the festival circuits so he's rarely in town on a weekend. They manage to see each other three weeks later and he's just as captivating as Meera remembers. Again, she can't quite work out what he thinks of her. Sometimes he's engaged, other times, his eyes scan the room as if he's looking for something better. She steps into overdrive, trying desperately to make him laugh, impress him with her music knowledge, keep him interested in what she's saying. She even bought a new T-shirt to wear that's edgier than her usual clothes.

They agree to meet again soon, but soon ends up being another three weeks. Three weeks in which Jay cancels and rearranges, and Meera loses her mind. It's a testing time for me, and the therapy, as I try to stay focused on Meera and not Jay (so as not to reveal that I know him, and also to help Meera to focus on herself). Privately, I'm not holding out much hope for Meera that Jay is going to commit to her like she so desperately wants.

She thinks of nothing but him, convinced he's the one. She talks about him to everyone who will listen, stalks his social media, spends hours researching places for their next date. When it finally arrives, Meera cannot contain herself. She grabs him outside the restaurant and they have another explosive kiss. Then, over the course of the meal, Jay retreats again, flipping from interested to distracted, giving no sense of why. Meera is anxious, unsure what these mixed signals mean. To her surprise, he invites her back to his and Meera is exhilarated again. She's been dreaming of what it might be like to sleep with him since their kiss. And it's every bit as intense and passionate as she imagined. Except afterwards Jay says he has an early start the next day and asks her to leave. She tries not to take it personally – even though she had grand plans to spend a lazy morning in bed, making love, ordering takeaway and eating it greedily together in bed. She leaves confused and even more infatuated than before.

Things continue in the same way, Jay cancelling dates and replying slowly to texts, then seeing each other and having a crazy, intense connection. It is both agony and bliss. On the one hand, Meera has never felt chemistry like it. On the other, Jay still hasn't made it clear how he feels. At any moment it seems like he might have lost interest. She spends hours waiting for messages, agonising to her friends, dropping the ball at work because she can't think about anything else. Just as Meera starts to think that maybe this isn't so good for her, Jay will send a sexy text and the whirlwind starts all over again. Meera has fallen hopelessly in love. The entire time, I wait for the inevitable.

Is intense chemistry a good thing?

Chemistry and attraction are not the same as love. We often have intense chemistry with people who trigger our childhood trauma – they remind us of something familiar and that familiarity feels erotic and exciting. Of course, you want to have sexual and emotional chemistry with your partner, but if things feel very up and down, burn brightly, then fizzle out, it might suggest that the early chemistry is really about fear.

This happens especially with people who make us feel rejected. Maybe they don't text back or initiate plans, they go days without communicating or shy away from commitment. This inconsistency triggers abandonment wounds, which triggers feelings of fear. Adrenaline and dopamine flood our system, which can make us feel excited and alive. We can get addicted to this feeling, which leads to obsession. We don't stop talking about them, they occupy all our thoughts, we start acting a little mad and do things to try to get their attention. It might feel very strong and very real, but those feelings are actually fear of rejection, which are usually coming from a deeper childhood wound of rejection.

It seems that Meera feels this intense passion for someone she doesn't know that well because he is triggering an early wound of rejection. Meera's parents split up when she was young. Her dad remarried quickly and had two kids with his new wife. When she spent time with him it was wonderful – he was playful and loving and present. Then, she'd go back to her mum's and her dad returned to his new family. Over time, her visits with her dad grew less and less frequent as he became preoccupied with his new family. Meera felt like she was second choice. Now she believes people are only caring and responsive some of the time. With men, this is the person she tends to go for – someone who blows hot and cold, who makes her feel special and adored, and then doesn't reply for a week – just like her dad.

From the start, she felt inferior and Jay's aloofness and cancelling of dates may only have made her feel more rejected and confused.

Fear of Rejection

Fear of rejection is something many of us struggle with. While it's normal to struggle with rejection we might be particularly sensitive if we've been rejected early on in our lives, because our minds are trying to protect us from it happening again. Each time we fear rejection it's likely to be coming from a past experience, which taught us that people who are supposed to love us hurt us. Inevitably the fear of rejection (when unhealed) ends up pushing people away and it becomes a self-fulfilling prophecy where we unconsciously create the very thing we feared happening, because it's what we feel we deserve.

Rejection wounds aren't always from direct rejection, such as being criticised or told off. Children can also feel rejected when they've been abandoned – for example, if a parent died or was generally absent. Rejection is also felt in the micro-moments: a parent preoccupied with their phone, emotionally disengaged or working a lot (even if done with good intentions, this absence can still be felt by the child as rejection).

– *EXERCISE* –

Reflect on your relationship to rejection. Where did you first experience rejection? Remember even if the rejection/abandonment wasn't intentional – like a parent returning to work early, or a family member dying, it can still feel like an abandonment to a child. Or perhaps your family were present but emotionally rejected you. Did you learn that you would be rejected for acting a certain way, like showing anger or sadness, or being too masculine or feminine? Were you made to feel wrong in some way?

How do you feel when you've been rejected? Where in your body does that show up? Is this similar to how you felt when rejected as a child?

Once we've connected to those painful feelings, we then have to soothe ourselves in the way we needed to be soothed as a child. Ask yourself what your child self would need to feel better when you're experiencing rejection. Rather than reaching out to someone else, what can YOU do to make yourself feel chosen and loved?

Why is fear sexy?

Fear can trigger sexual arousal in the body, which sets you on a rollercoaster of highs and lows. This happens when that person is similar to the people who hurt us when we were little. The chemistry and excitement we feel may actually be fear and terror that we're going to get hurt again in the same way.

This person reminds us of when our parents (for example) were inconsistent – maybe they were sometimes very loving but sometimes in a bad mood; maybe they were focused on their own needs and not ours, which made us feel rejected. That familiar rejection makes us want to do everything we can to stop it from happening again – hence the scheming and obsession. Our inner child is trying desperately not to feel rejected again. This desperation feels like intense chemistry. In the short-term, adrenaline kills pain, so when they choose us again the pain of rejection is soothed and it feels exhilarating and relieving.

Drama may feel fun and exciting, but it is not deep and safe love. If you're drawn to dramatic situations, there might be something you need to look at from your childhood relationships.

I want to be clear – sexual chemistry is not necessarily a red flag; it's a healthy need for a relationship. To figure out whether the intense chemistry is healthy or not, it is useful to look inwards. If the chemistry you are experiencing feels urgent and all-consuming, and comes with inconsistent behaviour or uncertainty about how they feel, this might be a sign that it is coming from an early wound, rather than from a genuine connection.

Tips if you feel intense chemistry with someone

- **Slow things down.** Chemistry is not connection. Try to really get to know this new person without rushing in and losing your sense of self.

- **Try to see whether this person is treating you in a similar way to how you've been treated before.** Is this a pattern?

- **How does it map onto your childhood relationships?** Generally, attraction is more intense with someone who triggers us. Get curious about what might be being triggered from your past.

- **Give people a chance to grow on you.** Deep love builds over time as you get to know each other better. Instead of choosing based on the chemistry from the first date, experiment with people who are different from your normal patterns and give feelings a chance to develop over time.

OBSESSION

Why Do We Get Obsessed with People Who Don't Want Us?

The worst happens. Meera sees a picture on Instagram of Jay on a date with a girl. She dives deep into the girl's social media. There's a picture of her and Jay smiling from a couple of months ago, back when Meera first met him. 'Date night with my man,' the caption reads.

I feel a hint of relief, even though it's hard to watch Meera descend into the pit of grief. She comes to our session in a pool of misery, shoulders hunched and sunken-eyed. All she can do is cry and talk about how amazing Jay was. She starts to grow anxious about her body. There's a pain in her chest – she's convinced it's a tumour, a heart attack, a death sentence. I wonder if what Meera might be dealing with is a broken heart.

She tells me, in forensic detail, everything that happened between them, over and over again. They have not spoken, though she's had ongoing conversations with him in her head. For Meera, this man lives on in her fantasies. She pictures the relationship they should have had. Meera imagines him coming back, bringing her back to life and taking away all the pain he has left in his absence.

As I listen, I hear how desperate, confused, possessed she is. The first thing I think is that these intense feelings must be about something more than just this man. Not that heartbreak isn't painful – of course it is – but I suspect that this is coming from a wound that was there long before he was. I ask, as I'm going to ask you now, to think about the model of relationships she's had in her life. What kind of expectations did her parents give her of what a relationship looks like, with each other and with themselves.

– *EXERCISE* –

I want you to think about the relationship between your parents. Are they together or apart? In what ways were they loving and in what ways were they distant? How did they show love, to each other and to you? Were they both emotionally and mentally present? Did you ever see them show physical affection? How did they talk to each other? Are there ways they showed contempt for each other? Are there ways they showed respect for each other? What did this teach you about relationships? How did this contribute to your expectations, your ability to give and receive love?

As you reflect on this, I want you to think about the relationships that were modelled down the generations: the relationships of your grandparents, aunts and uncles. All of these will form the blueprint for your understanding of what a relationship is, which creates expectations that you bring into new relationships.

It's not just your family relationships that shape your views, it's also your culture. Your race, class, gender, religion and sexuality will have sent you messages about what a relationship should be. What are your cultural expectations of a relationship? Are there rules or judgements about sex? Are there certain gender roles you carry? Is there shame about doing things differently from the norm? Even if you don't consciously agree with some of the cultural expectations you've absorbed, how might some of them have seeped into your blueprint of how a relationship should look?

This is important because we are each coming in with a blueprint for how relationships should be. The more we are aware of this blueprint, the more we might understand where our difficulties come from.

What's underneath?

Over several months, I try to get a sense of Meera outside of Jay – what are her interests, her desires, her identity – but every time we move away from Jay, she finds a way to veer back to him. I also gently (and sometimes clunkily) ask about her parents, but she shuts me down and steers the conversation back to men. I'm frustrated at having the same conversation about this guy and all the ways he still haunts her.

I guess that her obsession with men is a strategy to avoid feeling. She goes round and round with these thoughts, never really letting in any pain.

The obsession itself is tormenting, of course. It is all-consuming and, in its own way, very painful. But it's also very heady. What I mean by that is that it all takes place in the mind. We talk, think, draft texts, stalk Instagram profiles, conjure up hypothetical situations, imagine seeing them, have lengthy conversations. All the while, we're not really feeling.

It's a way to avoid the real pain, because the person is still with us in some way. We haven't lost them because we're keeping them alive in our mind.

Obsession with an ex is really a denial of loss. We don't want to let go. We don't want to grieve. Even if you never really had them, there's still the loss of the fantasy relationship you wished you could have.

There's also something about the rejection that drives us mad. In a brain imaging study by anthropologist Helen Fisher, they scanned fifteen people who had recently been rejected and showed them photos of the person who'd rejected them (not the most ideal post-heartbreak activity!)[14]. Looking at their past partner activated the brain areas involved in motivation and reward, as well as the dopamine system. The researchers took this to mean that romantic rejection is a 'goal-oriented motivation state rather than a specific emotion' and that their results are 'consistent with the hypothesis that romantic rejection is a specific form of addiction'. Basically, being rejected literally drives us to want them more. And this chase can be addictive. That's why 'playing hard to get' makes other people work harder. Now, please don't take this as an instruction to play hard to get – cat and mouse is really not a solid foundation for a healthy relationship.

The good news is that they also found the more time that had passed since the rejection, the less activity there was in those areas. This is basically neuroscientific evidence that time heals. It's a little like going cold turkey when abstaining from an addiction. The longer you withdraw, the less addicted and motivated to chase them you will feel.

But why is it that some of us chase the person who rejected us, and some move forward and look for someone who chooses them back? There may be many unconscious reasons, but here are three common ones:

1. Repeating patterns

The way Jay is treating Meera directly mirrors how things were with her dad – how he prioritised his new family after the divorce, making Meera feel second best. She'd yearn for his love, living off his presents and short visits as if they were keeping her alive in the gaps. Her obsession with being chosen and loved by Jay is a repetition of that childhood wish to be loved and chosen by her dad.

You may be thinking, 'Why do we go for people like our parents?' Well, we are drawn to what's familiar. Familiarity feels safe. Even if familiarity is people who abuse us like our parents did, people who are controlling like our mothers, or aloof like our fathers. It might not feel very nice to be in that kind of relationship, but as long as it's familiar our brain will often choose it.

One of my favourite Instagram quotes from the founder of online community Rising Woman, Sheleana Aiyana, is: 'We chase from our wounds, we choose from our worth.' Meera is chasing from a place of pain. She's trying to prove that she's lovable, because she was made to feel unimportant at times.

I think when we chase, we are acting from our wounded-child place. If you grew up with parents or siblings or a community who made you feel rejected in some way, you are likely to be attracted to people who make you feel this same way. Even though we know that those types of relationships bring us pain – something you might already be well aware of – your unconscious still sees people who meet your blueprint as normal and familiar. If we have a history of rejection, we expect rejection and therefore unconsciously attract situations that make us feel rejected.

2. Trying to write a different story

Another reason is that we're seeking a different ending to the original story that hurt us. The hurt child in you chooses familiar situations to the first, early wound in the hope that the outcome will be different this time.

Meera is choosing someone just like her distant father in the hope that this time she'll be able to make them love her.

Why do we do this? Freud thought that in these moments we are trying to gain mastery, but others believe that children are trying to redeem themselves[15]. Little Meera might have thought her dad was sometimes detached because she'd done something wrong – because she was insufficient, too much, unlovable. When Meera is drawn to people like her dad, she's trying to make them pick her so she can finally prove that she is worthy of love.

We repeat our patterns because we hope things will be different next time. Unfortunately, that is rarely the case. This is retriggering and why obsession and post-rejection pain can be so strong – it isn't just the hurt from that person we're feeling, but all the rejections that have come before them. It's the little children in us crying for their parents who didn't always show up in the way we needed.

3. Control

When someone rejects us, we are completely out of control. There's literally nothing we can do. Rather than accept that the person doesn't want us any more – which would come with lots of painful feelings we don't want to feel – we try to take back control.

All our plotting and thinking makes us feel like we're in control; if we just figure out the perfect thing to say or do, maybe we can get them back.

Anxiety is a way to feel in control of an uncontrollable situation, remember? (See page 61.) While there's nothing Meera can do to get this man back, by obsessing about him and plotting in her head, she feels some semblance of being able to stop the rejection from happening.

– EXERCISE –

I want you to think about your relationship patterns. If you could describe the type of person you tend to go for, what traits often come up? And no, I don't mean 'what's your type' in the aesthetic sense; it doesn't really matter what they look like. I want you to reflect on the key qualities and ways of communicating you're drawn to, and the situations that tend to unfold. Do you notice any patterns? Are there any similarities to your childhood relationships? Try to carefully think about the traits (healthy and unhealthy) you tend to be attracted to and whether they are familiar in some way.

How do we heal?

Slowly, as her obsession slightly wanes, Meera tells me how horrible it was after her parents divorced. One evening after school, she found her mum on the floor with a box of broken eggs, sobbing. 'He's found someone else! Someone prettier and younger. How can I – a frumpy old mum – compete with that? No wonder he left us.'

As Meera scooped up the eggs and set about making them a different dinner, it dawned on her that maybe she was the cause of the divorce, of her mum's unhappiness. Maybe her dad wouldn't have left if it wasn't for her. Now, in the present, Jay's ghosting triggers these feelings all over again – that she is to blame for people leaving.

I'm deeply saddened to hear this, but Meera still doesn't seem to feel anything. 'I just don't get how talking about the past is going to help,' she shrugs. I realise that maybe Meera is right in a way; all the feelings she might have had about the divorce and her parents are being projected onto this man. If she wants to talk exclusively about him, I'll have to meet her where she's at. So, I change tack and try to focus on how it felt when he went cold on her.

Meera says she felt sick. There was this sense of inevitability, as if she'd known it was going to happen all along. I ask if she can accept that he's gone. She says no, it's too painful. 'What if I start crying and never stop?'

It's a common fear, one I can reassure her does not happen. People always stop (at least in my experience). The fear is that crying would break you, that it would rip you open and you wouldn't be able to function. And maybe it will for a little while. In grief we take to our bed, we cry, we get angry, we don't eat or sleep or work. We have to feel safe in order to break down. We have to have space and time and support. It can be overwhelming, but this is a process that, for most people, has an end. If the loss is felt, the pain does subside.

Meera looks at me, tears in her eyes, and says, 'I have to accept I've lost him, don't I?' We both know she's not just talking about Jay. I nod, solemn but relieved that she's finally got there. She takes to her bed, she weeps, she lets her body mourn this man, and with it the divorce, her mum's fragility, her dad's new family.

Acceptance and grieving are the key to healing obsession. Acceptance is saying: this happened, it hurt, there's nothing I can do about it, so I'm going to write a new story. Meera needs to feel the pain, the loss, so she can let go of Jay, and the grief she feels towards her Dad, and choose from a place of awareness and self-worth.

The strategies I'm describing with Meera are for long-term healing. This takes a bit more time, and I recognise that you might want some things that work right now, so here are some more practical tools you can use alongside the longer-term work.

Tips if you're struggling with obsession

- **Stop feeding the obsession.** Stop bringing the person up in conversation or going over and over the stories. Think of it like a fire you're trying to let burn out. The more you talk about them, and to them, the more you're feeding the fire. Get a healthy distance and stop contact if you can. Being too close only feeds the obsession.

- **Learn to feel whole on your own so you don't feel you need them as much.** Refocus your energy on yourself, doing things you love and prioritising your pleasure, so you don't feel so dependent on them to be happy.

- **Let yourself grieve.** It's over, you don't have them any more, there's nothing you can do. Let go of control and let go of them, and allow whatever painful feelings come with that loss to move through you.

CHOOSING A PARTNER

Why Do 'Nice Guys' Feel Boring and 'Bad Guys' Feel Exciting?

Six months of mourning later and Meera feels ready to date again. She goes on a string of dates and comes to therapy each week to report back to me. Our sessions start to feel a bit like a glorified Hinge swipe. At one point she even gets her phone out to show me the lack of viable options. Most look perfectly nice to me, but her analysis is almost always the same – the men are too dull. He's sweet but dry, hot but not interesting, too keen, too nice. Not Jay enough.

Why is being too nice a problem? Why are we turned off by people who seem boring and stable?

There are a few potential reasons why we might struggle to be with people who commit and treat us well:

1. **Drama is addictive.** If we've grown up in chaotic home environments, we might not feel comfortable when things feel calm and slow. By choosing or creating situations that are intense and rejecting people who are too nice, we're repeating the chaos that feels familiar (and therefore safe).

2. **We don't feel we deserve to be treated well.** Our unconscious self seeks people who reinforce the way we feel about ourselves. If we're treated with love and respect, we'll choose people who love and respect us because we understand it's what we deserve. If we weren't loved in a healthy way, we may have learnt that this is what we deserve and seek that out in our adult relationships. Your choices in romance, friendships and your career are partially a reflection of how you feel about yourself – as well as influenced by your social status, class, education, race, etc. If 'nice' guys seem uninteresting, it might be because you don't feel you deserve to be loved.

3. **Fear of intimacy.** By pursuing someone emotionally unavailable, who treats us badly or can't commit, we are protecting ourselves from risking deep and vulnerable love. Choosing 'bad' guys means we don't have to depend on them and face all the fears that come with letting someone in. I'll talk more about this next.

Why do I keep choosing emotionally unavailable people?

It's important to understand that there's a difference between unavailability and emotional unavailability. If you go for people who are married or won't commit to you, you're chasing people who are simply unavailable. People who are emotionally unavailable are slightly harder to spot – they might want to be in a relationship, but they're afraid of intimacy. If you're in a relationship with someone who can't open up and you want things to be different, the best thing you can do is own your own fears of vulnerability and get working on yourself.

Emotional Availability

If you tend to choose people who aren't emotionally available, this is usually because you are afraid of intimacy yourself. Being vulnerable is risky. Many of us have grown up being told not to be too emotional or too sensitive. We may have been shamed or dismissed for opening up in the past. Protecting ourselves against vulnerability – by shutting people out or choosing people who shut us out – is a coping skill we learn as children that feels safer. The problem is, it doesn't serve us well as adults.

Instead of trying to change your partner and focusing your energy on getting them to open up, turn your attention inwards.

Jay, for instance, was desperate to fall in love, yet I think it's safe to say he was emotionally unavailable, because as soon as he realised the other person was imperfect, he would sabotage things. Jay found it easier to live in fantasy relationships and run when things got real, rather than risk real relationships with all the potential hurt that can come from them.

Meera, too, lived in a fantasy. Her fantasies were stuck in the past, with dreams of her ex finally coming back into her life. Clinging on to someone who is gone is also a form of emotional unavailability. By fantasising about her ex, Meera could protect herself from opening up and getting hurt all over again.

Situationships: why won't they commit?

Situationships by their very definition are relationships that remain undefined or lack commitment. Some of us stay in situationships for months, even years, wondering why on earth this person won't commit to us. This is the wrong question! The right question is: why are you entertaining someone who won't commit to you?

Don't worry, I've been stuck on this same question many times. Each time someone would protest at putting a label on things or avoid commitment, I would try desperately to understand what was wrong with this person. Did they have an avoidant attachment style or a traumatic childhood? Why were they so afraid of commitment and how could I convince them that they wanted to be with me? Maybe if I acted perfectly chilled and didn't ask for too much, or if I sent a funny enough message or did everything they asked, maybe *then* they'd want to be with me.

It took me going to therapy to realise that I was asking the wrong questions. I needed to understand what it was in me that was happy to accept crumbs. Why was I putting up with this? Why was I actively chasing people who were pushing me away?

I realised that, even though I would tell myself that I wanted a relationship and was always searching for one, deep down I was really scared of being in a committed adult relationship myself. It wasn't only the people I was chasing who had the issue with commitment; I was demonstrating that I was also afraid of commitment by staying in these situationships. It was a bit confusing at first – I was the one who wanted to get serious, who would have done anything to be with them, who was completely committed. But the relationship I wanted to be in with them was a fantasy. The reality was something casual, without much risk or intimacy. Holding on to the fantasy stopped me from having to be in a relationship. It was protecting me from all the fear that comes from finally letting someone in and relying on them.

– *EXERCISE* –

Reflect on why you might be choosing people who are closed. Were the adults in your life closed off from their feelings as a child? Are you repeating something familiar?

If we go with the idea that choosing someone emotionally unavailable is a way to protect yourself against the risk of intimacy, think about why vulnerability might feel scary for you. What are your experiences of being vulnerable in the past – has it been met with acceptance or rejection? Why might you need to protect yourself from getting too close to someone?

Letting ourselves depend upon, and love someone, is one of the bravest things a person can do. This is true for all forms of love. We are always risking the fact that the other person could leave at any time, or circumstances could take them away from us. This is why love can be so painful and terrifying for many. Letting someone in is threatening because we have no real control, which is why people close themselves off or cling on more tightly.

Bold, healthy love means to let someone in fully and also to accept that they may leave, while bearing all the fear and pain that comes with that (as well as all the lovely stuff too).

How can I become less emotionally unavailable?

GET CURIOUS: The important first step to becoming more emotionally available is to be aware – to identify that you are also avoiding intimacy and closeness. Even if you're the more anxiously attached one (we'll get to attachment styles next – see page 211), you are still likely to be scared of vulnerability and intimacy. So get curious with yourself about why that might be. You can't solve a problem unless you know what the problem is.

UNDERSTAND: Try to pay attention to the patterns in your relationships and learn from them. What triggers those fears? Notice when you want to pull away or close yourself off from people. If you keep choosing unavailable people, why might that be? What is it that might scare you about being close? And where do these fears come from? Can you track them back to anything in your childhood that taught you that being close is a risk? Try to give yourself space to work out what might have triggered you to protect yourself.

FEEL: Now that you've named your fears, you also have to feel them. Connect to your feelings without judging yourself, being as honest as you can about how scary it is to be intimate and close. Maybe you're very in touch with your desire for closeness, and feel frustrated at someone for denying you that. You might find yourself fixated on the other person and all the ways they're to blame. If so, bring your thoughts and feelings back to yourself. Do you want to be close and intimate but feel angry at the other person for pushing you away? Can you recognise that pursuing someone unavailable is really you denying yourself the closeness you crave?

ACT: It's not enough just to understand and connect to any fears of intimacy; you also have to do something differently within your relationships to stop yourself from acting on those fears. The best thing you can do is name them and communicate them to your partner, or even early on in the dating phase (set a precedent for good communication from the start!). Try to show your vulnerability and allow yourself to depend on them. If you're more anxiously attached in the relationship, this might look like being really honest about your fears of rejection and insecurity. If you're more avoidantly attached (see page 215), perhaps communicate that you're feeling the need for independence to feel safe, as well as any deeper feelings of fear that are causing you to pull away – that they might abandon or hurt you, for example.

REPEAT: You know the deal by now – this isn't going to change overnight; it's only going to change with work. Change happens in the small moments, in the difficult conversations, in the setting of boundaries, in the recognition of incompatibilities and polite rejection of situations that aren't right for you, in the owning of your own fears and attempts at sabotage. It might sound overwhelming or even frightening, but if you start small, you'll be on the road to change, hopefully without it seeming like too much.

Choose a partner who will help you to heal

Now you've focused on yourself, you can think about whether the partners you choose are hindering or helping you to be open or closed. An important step in building deep intimacy with someone is to choose someone who is (or is trying to be) emotionally available with you. If you continue to choose people who shut down or dismiss you and show no intention of working on this, it'll be hard to do the work yourself.

So if you're dating or considering a different partner, make sure you choose someone who shows signs of being emotionally available, or who is at least taking steps to become so.

Your choice of partner is a window into what needs healing. The traits you're drawn to are windows into your wounds. We go towards people who have both the light and shadow traits of our caregivers.

We have strong chemistry with people who mirror our childhood patterns. For example, if you had few boundaries as a child, you might be attracted to people with poor boundaries as an adult. You might also be attracted to the opposite – people with overly strong boundaries who give you the illusion of safety.

If your parents were sometimes very loving but sometimes very angry, you might be attracted to partners who blow hot and cold or have mood swings, or maybe you'll go for the opposite – someone who keeps all their feelings in – to protect yourself against anger. Whether we choose a mirror image or the opposite of our caregivers, our partners are typically coming from those early wounds. To start to heal and choose partners who are good for us, the first step is to pay attention to the type of person we're attracted to – they show us what needs healing.

Why do we go for people like our parents?

If we are treated with love and respect while we're growing up, we will understand that this is what we deserve. If not, we will constantly seek in others what we didn't have as young children. This constant seeking, this need to fulfil emotional voids, makes us vulnerable to falling into more destructive relationships.

When Meera's parents split up, her mum became highly anxious and not always present with Meera, so Meera had to step into more of a parent role. It's not a big-T trauma, but it's enough to make a small child feel dismissed and unimportant. Sometimes it not so simple as one trauma impacting us, but the ripple effects of the responses to trauma that also impact us as children. It seems that it's not just the feelings of abandonment by her dad triggered by Jay, but also the inconsistency of her mum, which motivated Meera to do everything she could to get Jay's attention, just as she used to do as a child.

So when Meera says the other men 'aren't Jay enough', I hear this as 'not Dad enough' or 'not Mum enough'. Meera is not interested in the nice and predictable options because all she knows are people who are inconsistent. The men who show up, who want a relationship, who really like her, are of no interest to the little girl inside Meera who is trying to finally make her dad choose her.

In order to grow and to break free from these patterns, it's important to become aware of your history and understand the origin of these sensations. Accept your history as part of who you are, process your emotions by feeling them fully and internalise them as lessons to redefine your beliefs about yourself.

So, how do I choose the 'right' partner?

As Meera continues to date, I grow exasperated. We go round and round the cycle – she either rejects men who seem lovely, or chases after someone like Jay, who never seems to be as into it as she is. The chemistry is intense, but she doesn't really get to know them, and they never know her. The rollercoaster ends and she's bereft once more, coming to me to pick up the pieces. I'm exhausted by the rigmarole of having the same conversation over and over again with no tangible change, just as Meera is.

One session, after I make another clunky link between the latest man she's pursuing and her father, she snaps. 'OK, I get it, I'm finding people like my dad, but how do I actually stop?'

Repetition Compulsion

This is one of the many theories of Freud's that is still relevant today – repetition compulsion is 'the desire to return to an earlier state of things'. When difficult aspects of relationships from childhood remain unprocessed, we seek out partners and friends who have similar dynamics to try to finally master them.

In adulthood this can manifest in different ways. If we grew up wishing our parents were more open and less dismissive, we might choose someone avoidant and dismissive and then spend years trying to get them into therapy. Or maybe we choose someone we feel we need to take care of, just as we felt we had to take care of our younger sibling or sick or fragile parent – unconsciously we are wishing that we could finally make that person better, or reaffirming our belief learnt in childhood that we need to be needed and of service in order to be loved.

We might consciously choose someone completely different, rebel against our parents entirely, but our unconscious unwittingly creates familiar situations without us even realising.

That's when I realise: I've been going round and round too. She understands she's going for men like her parents (I've harped on about it enough), but that isn't enough to change her. Frustrated and at the end of my therapeutic tether, I need to try something different. So I change tack. I stop talking to her intellectual brain, which now understands the problem, and instead address the vulnerable part of her that is stuck in this exhausting cycle.

In answer to her question, I reply, 'You grieve, not just for Jay, or the others, but for your dad, and for what your mum wasn't able to give you. You accept that your parents are never going to give you the kind of love and attention you crave.'

There's a full silence. The grief hangs thick in the air. Meera is fighting back tears and I decide to push her, to get us off this roundabout of intellectual understanding.

'I can see you're in pain, Meera. What would happen if you let yourself feel it?'

'It's too much,' she says, her voice quivering. 'It's too much.'

Except I can see from the way she chokes up that she is feeling it. Now, Meera has cried many times in my room, but this feels like a different sort of crying. A deeper, more honest crying. It seems that finally she's connecting to the real source of her sadness.

In the next session she tells me that she left last week and sobbed uncontrollably. She thought about herself as a child, remembered how she'd watch the door, waiting for her dad to come home, wondering what she could do to make everything go back to normal. How, after the divorce, her mum would have this glazed look in her eyes like she wasn't home – the same kind of look Jay would give. She remembers being intentionally naughty to get her to react, breaking things or throwing tantrums, just to get her attention.

She takes these memories into her next dates. When she gets that familiar feeling of intensity – if someone doesn't text back for days, dismisses her feelings or won't commit to plans – she thinks of that little girl. 'This isn't what that little girl deserved and it's not what I deserve,' she tells me proudly when she first ended things with someone who kept stringing her along.

It's not that Meera is no longer attracted to inconsistent men – she is. But she knows it won't make her happy, so she's actively making different choices. She gives more time to the consistent men, the ones who text back and are just as excited to see her as she is. She meets Liam. Liam is kind and funny and present. She doesn't want to rip his clothes off quite as much as she did with Jay, but she does want to talk to him, to know him and be known by him. When they kiss it's gentle and safe. He feels soft and reassuring. Meera finds herself opening up. She shares her dark and weird and silly thoughts with Liam, and encourages him to do the same. It's a different kind of love to the one she's known. She wants to be there for Liam, cook him nice meals, stroke his hair when he's stressed and hear about his day. It's in these mundanities, Meera realises, that peace is found.

Sometimes she misses the thrill of the chase, but she now understands how much more important it is to feel safe and loved. It is, she explains in our final session, a little unexciting sometimes. She smiles widely. Maybe that's how it's supposed to be.

Now that Meera has finally grieved the loss of her dad, and the lack of emotional presence of her mum and accepted that things were not her fault and that they will not change, she has started to break free from the anxious patterns she was stuck in. To make healthier relationship choices you must become aware of these patterns and shift the narrative of what you believe you deserve.

Things to look for in a 'healthy' partner

- You feel calm in their presence. Your nervous system isn't triggered by them in a way that puts you on edge. They feel safe and calm. It's even common to feel sleepy or tired when you're around someone who regulates you.
- They are consistent and their actions match their words.
- They are open and connect to their feelings. They don't dismiss yours and can tolerate difficult or emotional conversations.
- They have an understanding of their past and how it's affected them.
- There's lightness and play as well as an ability for seriousness.

It's important to say that if you struggle with relationships and have been let down deeply in your early life, you might struggle to feel safe and soothed by an emotionally healthy person immediately. It might take time and the repeated experience of not being let down that will create the security over time. It's the same in therapy – people don't feel completely safe with their therapists right away; it takes time to create trust. In the early stages, a secure partner can feel scary, but security is co-created within the relationship.

Section Three
In the Relationship

ATTACHMENT STYLES

How Do I Work on My Attachment Style?

Connor knows he wants Abby as soon as he sees her. She's dancing with her friends, in a blue satin dress, as her sandy hair swings, carefree, round her face. There's something gloriously sexy about the way she can't dance; her awkward movements are completely out of sync with the music, yet she dances with full enthusiasm anyway. He wants to be near her infectious energy. He slides over to her, and she meets his eyes with a wide smile. He charms her with his Galway accent, and they don't leave each other's side all night.

The first few months are a euphoric bubble of passion and romance. Things feel simple and light, as they so often do at the beginning.

The problems begin when things start to progress.

He's recently been made a manager at the bar where he works, which means more late nights and less time for Abby. Abby, on the other hand, is struggling to find work as a freelance writer, meaning she has a lot of time for Connor. Abby wants everything fast and Connor needs everything slower. She suggests moving in together after six months, which seems reasonable to her but is much too soon for him. He is barely ready to call her his girlfriend. Abby introduced Connor to her friends and family at the first chance she got; Connor hasn't even introduced her to his mum yet. 'Do you even want to be with me?' Abby asks, after Connor tells her he's going to renew the contract on his flat with his mates. He reassures her, again, that he does, but Abby isn't satisfied. It's important to Abby that they text frequently, otherwise she starts to doubt his feelings. She instructs Connor that he needs to text her more, which makes him want to text her less. He's irritated and starts hanging out with his friends more. He loves Abby, he really does, but his life is busy and he wants to use his days off to chill. Being around her is exhausting. It starts to feel like he has to take care of her, like she's burdening him with all her feelings. He complains to his friends that Abby is too clingy, too needy, too controlling. Abby complains to her friends that Connor is cold and aloof, emotionally unavailable, a commitment-phobe.

Abby can sense Connor's annoyance, and that he wants to spend less time with her, which only makes her more anxious. She tells him it's not enough; she needs to see him at least four times a week otherwise she thinks he'll forget about her. 'I'm your girlfriend,' she insists. 'You should want to see me all the time.'

Connor can feel the familiar tension creeping into his muscles. He wants to run. He wants to shout, 'Back off – let me breathe!' He goes into a different room, trying to get some space. Abby stands in the kitchen, alone and rejected. Anxiety bubbles through her chest. Why doesn't he love her? He clearly doesn't love her. Desperate, she follows him into the bedroom and begs him to talk to her.

Can you see how Abby and Connor have conflicting needs? Abby needs closeness to feel safe, Connor needs space. This is such a common pattern of relationships – you may recognise yourself in either Abby or Connor. If this sounds somewhat familiar, your attachment needs might be playing a bigger part in your relationships than you realise.

What is attachment theory?

Attachment theory was introduced by psychologist John Bowlby in 1969[16] and explains how our early relationships with our caregivers create our expectations for how we think relationships should be. Babies are born with a need for closeness so that they will survive. They will adapt to how their parents react to them to keep the bond and increase their chances of survival. Our sense of self and relationships is based on how our parents respond to us as children, and how we adapted to their responses.

So, if a parent leaves, is violent, ignores us, is unpredictable, too controlling or highly anxious themselves, it's a threat to that child's entire life. This is why early relational trauma affects us for our whole life – because it's so impactful on those early years of development.

Conversations on attachment theory have exploded since 2020. It feels like everyone is taking the test to see what their attachment style is or diagnosing their partners so they can blame all their problems on their partner's attachment style (I've been there too, believe me!). Or, maybe, like Connor and Abby, you haven't thought about your relationships too deeply, but you've noticed you often end up in the same patterns of conflict.

Attachment theory, when used appropriately, can be a really helpful tool to enable us to understand what's going on in our relationships. It's something I find useful to understand myself, my own relationships and the work with my patients. In this chapter I'm going to give you an overview of each attachment style, how it's formed and how it shows up in adult relationships so you can start to think about how this might be affecting you and your relationships.

How does each attachment style develop?

Inside all of us is an attachment alarm. As babies, separation from our parents is terrifying, because without them we die. If there is too much distance, the attachment alarm will go off. This applies not only to physical separateness, but also emotional separateness. If a parent is detached, stressed, anxious, cold or distracted, a baby senses that and the attachment alarm will go off. Babies tend to cry or do something to get their parents' attention. If the parents respond and attune to their child's feelings, babies learn that their parents are there and feel safe again. When a caregiver is reliable and present, they become what's called a secure base. Because the child knows they have their parents to come back to for protection and reassurance, they are then more confident to explore and play, taking more risks as they know their parent will be there for them when they return. If they don't respond, or respond inconsistently, insecure attachment develops. There are two main ways that babies respond when their parents aren't responsive: anxiety or avoidance. Either they cling and ask for attention or shut down and pull away.

Secure attachment: children feel confident and are able to be soothed. They're upset when they're separated from their parents and able to be comforted by them. When their parents are around they feel soothed and safe enough to explore.

Anxious attachment: babies become quite anxious, cry more loudly, scream and try to get their parents' attention. If that works, babies learn that they need to cling and cry to get attention.

Avoidant attachment: if the strategy doesn't work, the baby will learn to stop crying altogether and instead shut down – because it's simply less painful to stop crying than it is to cry and have no-one come. They will struggle to open up and connect deeply with others as they've learnt to pull away and rely on themselves to feel safe. Because we're wired to develop in ways our parents want us to and we read the unconscious messages we're taught, we might also learn that self-reliance is encouraged by getting praised for not crying or making a fuss.

Disorganised/fearful attachment: disorganised attachment (or fearful) is a combination of anxious and avoidant styles. Sometimes they feel fearful of rejection and cling, while other times they pull away and need space. This generally forms when children are afraid of their caregivers, so when the parent is more abusive. They need love and care, but they're also afraid of the parent, and fear makes them flip between both anxious and avoidant styles – either clinging or pushing away. This is the most damaging form of attachment because there is no safe place to go, which is why strategies such as addictions (which can act as substitute caregivers that can be relied on) are much more likely. While they can help a child adapt to a frightening situation in early life, they lead to significant problems in adulthood.

Before you start diagnosing yourself, think about how your parents responded to you:

- Were they mostly there, or were they sometimes there and sometimes not? Not just in terms of physical needs, but for your emotions too.
- Did you trust them to be there?
- Were they able to soothe you?
- Do you feel comfortable opening up to them? Were you encouraged to voice your needs and express your vulnerability?
- Did you ever feel afraid of them?
- Who did you turn to for care when you were scared/upset/sad? If it wasn't a parent, ask yourself why. If it was one parent and not the other, think about your relationship with the parent you didn't seek care from versus the one you did.

How does each attachment style show up in adult relationships?

Bowlby believed that our attachment style affects us from 'the cradle to the grave', and extensive research has backed this up. Our attachment style as a child determines the type of relationships we have as adults, how we deal with conflict, our expectations of love and our attitudes to sex, as well as a whole host of other factors, such as self-esteem, overall mental health, resilience, our ability to deal with stress, and school and career outcomes.

As adults, we still have this attachment alarm, and it is particularly triggered by romantic relationships. When we feel safe and secure, our attachment alarm stays quiet. When we feel insecure, the attachment alarm is activated, usually by someone either pulling away (instigating anxious attachment) or someone getting too close (instigating avoidant attachment). With disorganised attachment, this can be triggered by someone being too close, inconsistent or even secure – it might feel very scary to have someone there to rely upon if your early experiences of relationships were full of fear.

Secure attachment: someone with a secure attachment is able to give and receive love. They are comfortable opening up to others and don't shy away from commitment and intimacy. They feel safe in relationships, meaning they can get close and take space when needed. They develop an identity of someone who is worthy of love and care. This will be their more typical way of being, but no one is 100 per cent secure all of the time – we all have insecurities and insecure parts of us, and our attachment alarms can all be activated by insecurely attached people.

Anxious attachment: people with an anxious attachment feel insecure in love and intimacy. They feel very anxious and sensitive to rejection, tend to need lots of reassurance and struggle with distance or separation. They have difficulty regulating their own feelings and need others to soothe them rather than being able to soothe themselves. They might become clingy, controlling and demanding.

Avoidant attachment: people with an avoidant attachment style will struggle with closeness. They feel very independent and tend to pull away from commitment or intimacy. They do not trust others, so they keep themselves safe by keeping other people at a distance. They also avoid difficult or painful feelings, and deny their needs for connection, instead projecting all their neediness onto other people.

Disorganised/fearful attachment: They both want and fear romantic relationships. So they seek out relationships but have trouble trusting and depending on people. They struggle to regulate their feelings and avoid relying on people for fear of getting hurt, or they over-rely on people and set themselves up for the very things they fear most: abandonment and rejection.

– *EXERCISE* –

As you start to reflect on these things, you might notice some patterns in your relationships, and some potentially common issues. What is your role? Are you highly independent and always helping others? Are you often needing others to make you feel better and can't function well on your own? Are you often the peacekeeper or the one starting the conflict? Examine your role in relationships and you will start to understand yourself.

It's important to understand that different attachment styles can be brought out by different people. In the past, when I've been in relationships with very avoidant people, I've moved more towards being anxious. When I've been with very anxious people, I've moved towards avoidant. That being said, most of us will tend to lean more heavily towards one attachment style. But don't be too confused if you don't fit neatly into one box – I'd encourage you to hold your attachment style lightly and notice when different people's behaviours trigger different responses.

NB Attachment happens between friends, colleagues and family members too, not just in romantic relationships. Because romantic relationships tend to be more intimate – like our child–parent relationships – attachment patterns tend to be more pronounced in that context, but they are at play in all relationships.

The anxious–avoidant cycle

Connor has an avoidant attachment, while Abby has an anxious attachment. It tends to be common that people with these attachment styles end up in relationships together. There is something almost magnetic about the two, where one's avoidance balances out the other's anxiety.

However, without proper communication and some self-awareness from both partners, this doesn't usually end well. Like Connor and Abby, the avoidant partner triggers all of the anxiously attached person's insecurities – they experience the withdrawal and pulling away as proof that their partner is rejecting them. Then the anxious person pushes their partner to open up and to come in closer, which only makes the avoidant person disconnect even further to protect themselves from this closeness, which exacerbates the anxious attachment even further.

How do you get out of this vicious cycle of conflicting needs?

We *can* change our attachment style, but it isn't always easy. We will always revert to our underlying attachment style at times of threat. Still, even without completely changing our attachment style, we can still transform our relationships by understanding our own and our partner's attachment insecurities.

First, it's important to know that the other person's reactions are *not always about you*. Connor withdraws because closeness feels frightening and he must protect himself (though he's probably not conscious of this), and Abby clings because space feels frightening to her.

A common problem I see in this dynamic is that it always feels like the other person's fault. And I've done this myself many times – blaming the relationship issues on the other person and believing that if they could just change their attachment style, everything would be fixed. This strategy never worked because I was in denial about my own attachment style and my reasons for staying with people who were consistently triggering my attachment alarm.

Avoidant–anxious relationships aren't typically one-sided – attachment styles interact with each other and exacerbate the opposing response. Abby would be happy if only Connor would open up, and Connor would be happy if only Abby would stop being so controlling. What is often happening is that one partner is projecting onto the other.

Projection

Projection is one of the most important concepts I wish everyone understood. One of the ways we escape our unconscious feelings and parts of ourselves is by projecting the things we don't like about ourselves onto other people. When we disown parts of ourselves (that we unconsciously think are unacceptable or shameful), we attribute them to others. These are mostly unpleasant, negative qualities, but it can also happen with positive qualities we don't recognise in ourselves – maybe we're obsessed with how beautiful other people are but are unable to recognise our own beauty. Have you ever felt instantly annoyed at someone's behaviour for no real reason? Chances are you're projecting that part of yourself onto them. Most of us don't realise just how much we're projecting onto others.

This is what people mean when they say 'relationships hold up a mirror' to ourselves: we see others not as they are, but as *we* are. When we're judgemental or critical of others, we're really being judgemental and critical of that part of ourselves.

We tend to choose partners who have traits we are denying in ourselves. This happens in so many relationships. Anxious–avoidant attachment dynamics are a classic case of this. The avoidant person is in complete denial of their neediness and fear of being left or let down. They feel completely independent, as if they don't need people at all. Then they choose relationships where the other person appears very needy, very afraid and vulnerable. They can feel like the non-needy ones because the anxious partner is carrying their need for them.

It's the same on the flip side. Anxiously attached people might project their emotional unavailability, their own fears of closeness, onto the avoidant person. Remember, both parties are afraid of intimacy. Both blame the other – if only they were less needy, or less closed off, the relationship would be fine.

I was struggling to give you a personal example of how I project, so I asked someone close to me for an example and they laughed and replied immediately: 'It's obvious, you project your vulnerability and neediness onto Albie.' Albie is my dog. He's the one who wants constant hugs and affection, he's the one who's needy. I'm the independent human who's totally fine on my own. Then he decides to exert his independence by sitting on the opposite side of the sofa and I feel outraged and demand he cuddle me instantly. Of course, it's really me who wants love and affection, but it's safer to put that onto Albie rather than own my own needs.

– *EXERCISE* –

Think of something that really annoys you in other people. Maybe you hate it when people complain a lot, or talk too much about themselves, or are overly needy. This is usually the part of ourselves we do not accept. Try to notice patterns in the way you judge others. What are the traits you find intolerable? In what ways might you have some of those traits? What stories are you telling yourself about them? Do you believe it's bad to talk too much about yourself or be needy? Are you denying your own desire to take up space or to depend on other people?

Examples of projection

- 'You clearly fancy them': being convinced someone will cheat when it's you who may be attracted to someone else or unsure about the relationship.
- 'That's disgusting': feeling disgusted about something is often a reflection of hidden shame. People respond this way to sex or homosexuality, for example, which is probably just their own shame and insecurities projected onto others.
- 'They're so needy': someone who declares everyone else is needy might be denying their own neediness.
- 'X is so annoying/ugly/lame/fat': often we project our own insecurities onto others by criticising them. Really, we're being critical of ourselves.

- 'X clearly doesn't like me': it may be you who doesn't like them, or yourself, but you defend against this feeling by projecting it onto the other person.
- 'Everyone here is making me uncomfortable': it might be you who feels uncomfortable, but you experience the problem as being caused by other people.

It seems as though Connor is projecting his own neediness and vulnerability onto Abby, believing that he is independent and without needs, while she is the needy and weak one. Abby might also be projecting her fear of intimacy onto Connor. She blames all this on Connor, feeling that he is the one preventing them from being close. Yet she is choosing someone who is keeping her at arm's length (remember, if you're in a relationship with someone emotionally unavailable, you may also be emotionally unavailable).

It's important not to get drawn into the (often very convincing) narrative that the other is to blame, and to explore the role each of you plays in perpetuating this cycle.

STOP!

If you've spent this chapter trying to understand your partner and their attachment style, stop and re-read it with the focus on yourself. Think about Connor and Abby – they both blame each other for being too clingy or too distant, without understanding their part in the relationship. The best thing we can do to improve our relationships is to take the blame off our partners and shift the accountability onto ourselves.

What helps Connor and Abby?

Connor and Abby do not want to break up. Instead, Abby convinces Connor to go to therapy.

At first, he uses the sessions to complain about Abby. Connor strongly believes that Abby is the problem, and he's convincing. I start to agree that Abby is needy and clingy, that if she would just be less anxious, he wouldn't be so avoidant.

That is until I start to feel needy and clingy myself.

His avoidance is palpable. He turns anything serious into a joke. When I attempt to get close to him, having moments of connection or vulnerability, he seizes up, visibly tenses and changes the subject. He cancels sessions, tells me he can't see himself doing this for long, always one foot out of the door. I start to worry that he won't come back, that every session will be his last. 'Now I've become the needy one,' I say to my supervisor, only half joking.

I wonder if this is how Abby feels: that Connor isn't fully in, that he might leave at any moment. No wonder she's anxious. Now, I'm not saying Connor is to blame either – I think people with an avoidant attachment are often demonised online, but it's important to remember that this is a dynamic that is created by two people. Still, until Connor is able to take his hand off the doorknob, I doubt Abby will ever feel secure in the relationship.

I start to steer the conversation away from Abby and on to his avoidance. 'What is it like when Abby tries to share her feelings with you?'

'It makes me cringe, like, just kind of shut down.'

'What's cringey about emotions?'

'I dunno, I just feel annoyed by them.' There's a story here, the rest of the iceberg to uncover.

Connor's family never spoke about feelings; they were a keep-calm-and-carry-on type of family, the kind who mocked sentimentality and kept all their vulnerabilities to themselves. His dad would laugh when Connor showed any kind of sensitivity, humiliated him for crying and being 'too soft'. After the age of five, his dad stopped hugging him – you're too old for all that, he would say. Connor learnt to stifle any attempts at closeness, burying his deep need for tenderness and love so his dad couldn't see it. Eventually, he got so used to hiding it that it became invisible to him too.

Now he feels humiliated at the very prospect of showing any feeling or expressing a need. He projects his fears of vulnerability onto others, seeing them as weak for daring to express themselves. I realise that the way I am feeling with Connor – anxious about being rejected, too emotional and sensitive – is probably the way he was made to feel by his dad. My job is to help Connor own that part of himself, so he can stop pushing away the things he probably desperately wants underneath.

'Have you ever thought,' I ask Connor, 'that Abby isn't as needy as you think? That maybe you also have needs? That maybe you want to be loved just as much as she does?'

He scoffs. 'Nah, I'm independent. I don't need people like she does.'

'We all have needs, Connor. What about that little boy who wanted a hug from his dad?'

He stares at the wall. 'Yeah, it was all I wanted from him.' The words catch in his throat. 'But I'm not a kid any more.'

'Maybe not, but adults need hugs too.'

Connor rolls his eyes at me, as he often does, and makes a joke about the Irish having Guinness to keep them warm at night.

The conversation moves on, but something has registered.

The next session, Connor announces that he is going to stop therapy. 'I felt you were a little more vulnerable with me last week,' I said – trying to stay calm and resist the desire to anxiously cling on – 'I wonder if your impulse to leave is connected to that.'

'What, like I'm running away?'

I raise my eyebrows in question.

'I guess I do have form for that,' he says.

Slowly he's starting to be a little more reflective. The vulnerability and need for intimacy that has been unconscious for so long is starting to come to the surface.

As therapy progresses Connor starts to admit he is afraid – afraid of showing his feelings, afraid of getting too close to someone in case they humiliate him – or worse, leave.

And, though it is immensely difficult to get there, he admits all of this to Abby.

He experiments with telling her how he feels, pushing through the urge to shut down. He explains how scary feelings are, how deep down he's terrified that if he opens up, she'll leave. 'That's why I need a bit of space. It's nothing to do with you. Emotions just feel shameful to me, but it is something I want to get better at,' he explains.

'So we're both scared the other one will leave?' Abby asks. Connor nods, and notices how good and scary it feels to be seen like this.

With Connor opening up, Abby admits that her anxious eruptions and controlling behaviour might be a way to get

Connor's attention. When she feels shut out, she worries he's forgotten about her or stopped loving her. The crying and the anxiety might be a way to get his love and care. It doesn't work, of course; it only seems to push Connor away.

Together they try to think about what they can each do differently – Connor to share his feelings and own his needs, and Abby to respect his need for space while expressing her need for attention and care from a more regulated place of independence.

Abby grins and they hug, both relieved to have shared something of themselves, to have done something differently from their usual push and pull. It's not the end of their struggles – Abby will find herself erupting again and Connor will pull away – but they will learn to deal with it differently. As Connor is increasingly able to come closer and open up, if feels safer for Abby to back off and soothe herself, and soon they'll find they're sharing more of themselves than they ever knew possible, talking into the middle of the night as if they're just meeting each other for the first time. And, in a way, they are.

Finding someone to do the work with

One of the reasons Connor and Abby were able to start to repair their anxious–avoidant dynamic is because both were prepared to work on themselves. It's very hard to do if only one of you is committed to doing the work. It might take one party to get the ball rolling, and usually that's going to be the more anxiously attached person (avoidants don't tend to seek out therapy as readily). But if you're trying to work on yourself, open up to the other person, take accountability and shift your patterns, your relationship is unlikely to change unless they are doing it too (though of course your change will hopefully have a positive effect on them).

If they are unwilling, or say they will but never do, ask yourself this: is this the right relationship for you? Be honest with yourself. Are there any patterns from childhood that you might be re-enacting in this dynamic? Are you holding on to a fantasy of this person changing, rather than the reality of who they are?

If you and your partner are both willing to reflect on these things and make changes, then you're halfway there. There's nothing I love to see more than two people committed to understanding themselves so they can heal their relationship together. Whether it lasts in the long-term or not, you can learn so much from a dynamic where you both tentatively dare to take the risk of vulnerability together.

Changing your attachment style is about creating safety and security in both yourself and your relationship. It's a gradual and partial process, rather than complete and black and white (i.e. one day I'm insecurely attached, the next I'm securely attached). Sometimes it's about creating a secure relationship together, which actually involves understanding, accepting and living with your attachment style and your partner's, so the relationship becomes one of secure attachment even while each partner has their own attachment style within it.

To do this it's important to recognise your triggers and patterns, then to try to shift your response when you're triggered. When your attachment alarm is going off, it tells you to either cling and seek reassurance or pull away and withdraw, or both. Healing your attachment style is about responding differently to that alarm, being understanding of and compassionate to the insecure part of you (your child part) and creating safety within yourself.

Tips for what to do when your attachment alarm is activated

- **First, recognise it's activated.** If you have the desire to cling or to pull away, or both, notice this desire and try to get some distance from it by taking a moment rather than acting on it straight away.

- **Think back to childhood** and other times when you felt these feelings before. Try to use this understanding to recognise that your attachment alarm is ringing at maximum strength and that it relates to early trauma rather than the real situation now. You can use this understanding to soothe that child inside.

- **Before you take action** (by clinging or withdrawing), try to self-soothe, making yourself feel calm and safe. If you tend to need others to soothe you, try to find ways to soothe yourself. If you tend to shut down, try to challenge yourself to open up and let yourself depend on someone else. Reassure yourself that you are safe. You are an adult and you do not need this person to survive in that moment. What can you do to regulate yourself?

- **Communicate with your partner.** Try to take accountability for your reactions rather than blaming your partner for triggering you. Express how you feel so they can recognise your needs and respond to them. Be as vulnerable and open as possible.

- **Allow yourself to feel (and communicate) the fear** of depending on someone. It's terrifying, and that's OK. All attachment styles have a deep fear of relying on someone, even for secure people relying on someone can feel scary. Rather than acting on it, let yourself feel that fear – the same fear you would have felt as a small child with parents or caregivers you couldn't fully rely on.

If you saw yourself or your partner in one of these attachment styles and want to learn more, I'd recommend the book *Attached* by Dr Amir Levine and Dr Rachel Heller, which takes a deeper dive into how attachment styles form, how they affect our relationships and how they can be changed.

CO-DEPENDENCY, BOUNDARIES AND PEOPLE-PLEASING

Why Do I Lose Myself in Relationships?

Soon into our work together, Kelley (the art student who struggled with anxiety and boundaries) falls in love. I get a text from her the day before our session. 'I HAVE NEWS.' She arrives early, bounds into the room and, before either of us has sat down, announces proudly that she has met someone.

I follow her new relationship like it's a Hollywood romcom, because that's how Kelley presents it. Trish is the most beautiful woman she's ever seen. She's hilarious and fun, they spend their time either laughing in bed or out dancing together. They take it in turns to surprise each other with breakfast in the mornings, and within weeks they're spending every night together. Suddenly every story or anecdote involves Trish, as if she's never existed without her.

Yet, despite hearing everything about this woman, there's something about Trish I can't quite grasp, as if she's this fictitious character without any depth. Kelley's idealisation of her makes the whole relationship feel slightly unreal. Where are Trish's imperfections, her flaws and problems? And, more importantly, why can't Kelley see them? It's common to see someone with rose-tinted glasses at the beginning, so I tell myself to stop being cynical and wait to see how things unfold.

And they unfold quickly. Within three months Trish has moved in. I mention how fast things are going to Kelley and she jokes that this is just how lesbians are, which shuts down any curiosity about what's going on. Still, I try to suspend my concern because Kelley really does seem happy.

Cracks start to appear by the summer. On a night out, Trish got sloppy drunk and started insulting Kelley's friends. It took two hours to get Trish home because she refused to get in the cab. Trish spent the next day guilt-ridden in bed, making Kelley promise she wasn't mad. She wasn't, she assures me, though all I can see are the way her fingers twist into each other as she says it, her body betraying her words. It's a one-off, she tells me, and herself.

Except it isn't. It is, in fact, the beginning of a slippery pattern of co-dependency. Trish gets drunk and Kelley takes care of her, then Trish feels depressed and guilty, and Kelley has to take care of her again, all the while pushing her own feelings aside.

As their relationship continues, Kelley's world starts to get smaller. She sees less of her friends, stops going to the art exhibitions she loves because Trish needs her at home, paints less because Trish is more interested in going out for dinners and drinking. The therapy is equally taken over by Trish. Kelley wants to find a way to help her, which might sound perfectly healthy, except that she becomes preoccupied, trying everything she can to convince Trish to get therapy, to stop drinking, to make her better. What transpires, as it often does in these kinds of relationships, is that the more Kelley helps, the worse Trish gets.

Her people-pleasing manifests in sex too. Kelley doesn't like to take up too much space in bed, so she never asks for what she needs. She focuses on Trish, never actually orgasming herself. She tells me she likes it this way; she's much more comfortable being the giver than the receiver. My alarm goes off again. Where are Kelley's desires? What about Kelley's satisfaction? She has needs too, but they seem to get cast aside to fulfil Trish's.

I point out to Kelley that we almost never talk about her. She laughs and says, 'Talking about Trish *is* talking about me.' I don't laugh with her because what she's telling me isn't funny at all. Kelley has become well and truly enmeshed with Trish – where she feels that they are one and the same. Slowly, Trish has started to eclipse her. It reminds me of the lack of boundaries Kelley has with her mum, as if they're one person. It seems to me that Kelley and Trish have become co-dependent.

What is co-dependency?

Healthy relationships are mostly balanced and equal. They have a reciprocal nature – 'sometimes I care for you, other times you care for me'. Co-dependent relationships are one-sided. One person does most of the giving and sacrificing, while the other does the taking. Often this looks like someone who is overly dependent, who is the 'needy' one, and someone who abandons themselves to meet the other's needs. This is the part of co-dependency that I think is often misunderstood. A lot of people think it is about spending lots of time together or both partners over-relying on one another, when really it's about an imbalance.

In a co-dependent relationship, each person unconsciously uses the other to play out their wounds. One person may lose themselves and abandon their needs, while the other uses and exploits the other to fulfil their needs. It's an enmeshed relationship where you lose your sense of independence. Co-dependency is a blurring of edges. There's a sense that you don't know where they start and you begin, which makes the bond even stronger and the relationship harder to leave, because you feel like you can't exist without the other.

Enmeshment

Enmeshment is a relationship with merged boundaries, where you don't know where the other person ends and you begin. You're expected to think, feel and believe the same way as the other person, almost becoming one. This makes it difficult to feel separate and stops true independence. If this characterises a parent–child relationship, it can make it hard for the child to move on from their family and form independent adult relationships. If you fantasise about people without actually being in serious relationships and have very close relationships with your family, you might be sabotaging your relationships because you don't actually want to grow up and separate from your parents.

You might be the one to abandon yourself to a relationship because you feel responsible for the other person's feelings and sacrifice your own needs to meet theirs. This goes hand in hand with people-pleasing. Because you feel responsible for the other person, you might neglect yourself and find it hard to set boundaries, say no and engage in conflict.

On the other side, you may be quite demanding and controlling, and find it hard to compromise. Perhaps you tend to blame other people for your feelings and see it as their responsibility to make you happy. On the more extreme end this can look like narcissistic abuse or coercive control – relationships where one partner is (often unconsciously) using their partner to get what they want.

Signs of co-dependency

- Abandoning your needs and desires.
- Feeling responsible for other people's feelings.
- Taking the blame or apologising to keep the peace.
- Needing approval and validation from others.
- Needing control.
- Often being in the carer role in a relationship.
- Avoiding conflict.
- Doing things you don't want to do to make others happy.
- Difficulty connecting to, and showing, feelings.
- Idealising other people.
- Low self-esteem and deep fears of rejection.

Why do we form co-dependent relationships?

In a co-dependent relationship, one person is often the 'needy' one and the other the fixer. This is a split of vulnerability and responsibility. All the vulnerability gets projected onto the needy one, which makes the fixer resentful at having to drop everything for this person, yet all the while the fixer's own vulnerability is being denied. Meanwhile the needy person has given up their sense of responsibility and agency to care for themselves, making them feel dependent on the other to help them.

As Kelley complains about Trish, she doesn't recognise the ways in which she is infantilising her and contributing to her dependent, needy state. She feels such a sense of responsibility to help Trish that she's actually disempowering her. It's as if Trish is a child, incapable of helping herself, though I'm not sure this is the reality. I suspect that Trish has fallen into the child role, while Kelley has taken up the role of the parent.

When you enter a co-dependent relationship, you're often modelling the kind of relationships you had in childhood. If a parent was particularly controlling or narcissistic, you might not have developed a strong sense of your own self and your own needs. Perhaps you were in a carer role as a kid, with your parents or siblings, and you learnt to feel valued by looking after people. Maybe you were shouted at, given the silent treatment or abused in some way, which made you terrified of conflict, so you learnt to people please as a way to keep them happy. Perhaps your family was enmeshed, so you felt you couldn't have boundaries or be too different from them.

Enmeshment might sound positive – we all want to be close to our parents, right? – but it shouldn't be confused with healthy closeness. Being too close can create an unhealthy dependence where your family member is using you to meet their emotional needs so you can't become yourself. Kelley was very close to her mum, but in a way that lacked boundaries and healthy separation, creating a tendency for Kelley to become overly dependent on people and lose her identity in relationships.

Enmeshment creates adults who:

- feel overly responsible for other people's feelings.
- prioritise the needs of others over their own.
- struggle with boundaries.
- act as the parent, trying to fix everyone.
- act as the perpetual child, never growing up and always looking for someone to take care of them.
- feel excessively guilty, as if they've done something wrong all the time.
- don't know or respect their own feelings and needs.
- can't tolerate differences between them and their partners or friends.

Enmeshment creates a kind of arrested development, where you don't quite grow up because you're still not independent. In my experience, this can have two effects on our relationships: we fantasise about relationships but never actually engage in them, or we enter into relationships that are lacking boundaries and are equally enmeshed.

How do you move on from your parents?

Emotionally separating from parents is one of the hardest things people struggle with in therapy. It's different for everyone, but psychologically moving away from the comfort of a close family is hard work. It's also the only way to feel free.

Emotional separation from your parents is very healthy. It's why teenagers suddenly start prioritising their friends and telling their parents that they hate them. If your teenager does this, or you did this as a teen, it's actually a healthy sign that they are separating into their own person with their own ideas and identity. It doesn't mean you can't still have a close and loving relationship with them, but you may need to separate first, learn to become your own person, so that you can have a person-to-person relationship with your parents, rather than stay stuck in a child–parent merger.

When I say separate, I don't mean with distance necessarily. Someone can be halfway around the world and still emotionally intertwined with their parents.

Separation is terrifying if we feel our parents can't handle it. They might need us to be just like them, feeling threatened by us being too different. We're aware of that threat and worry that we'll upset them, that they won't like us if we're different from them. But in staying attached we give up our independence and sense of self as a whole person.

If you don't have a relationship with your parents, or if they aren't alive any more, you can still separate from them emotionally; it's more of an internal process than anything.

Separating from our parents can also happen through emotionally separating from our adult partners, who often become our surrogate parents. Learning to have boundaries and become more independent in our adult relationships is a way to become more separate from the parent–child dynamic within co-dependent romantic relationships.

Self-abandonment

Even if you did grow up in a loving and stable home, you may have learnt that you were good if you did what your parents wanted, and bad if you did what they didn't want. So as adults we still believe that to be loved and accepted by others, we have to do what they want, even if we don't want to.

Whatever the reason, you will have been taught at some point that you were responsible for other people, that your needs and feelings were not as important as theirs. If we put other people's needs first from such a young age, we might not be aware of our own feelings, needs, desires and boundaries. Being so fixated on others leads us to becoming completely out of touch with ourselves – this is self-abandonment.

It seems at first that Kelley is giving up her needs willingly: she wants to drop everything to help Trish; she wants to cancel the exhibitions so she can spend time with her – it's only me who sees any of this as problematic.

Except every time she talks about taking care of Trish, or giving something up, she wrings her fingers around each other.

'You seem a little annoyed,' I suggest, nodding to her fingers.

Kelley groans. 'OK, fine, yeah, it's a bit annoying. It's like Trish is so fragile that I can't do anything I want. It's never about me.'

It seems, as so often happens when someone is self-abandoning or people-pleasing, that some resentment towards Trish has trickled in.

Resentment

People-pleasing and co-dependency rarely exist without resentment. Often, if our boundaries have been violated, we will have a physical feeling of discomfort.

Any people pleaser will know the bitterness that comes with doing something they don't want to do. Even though you haven't said no (probably because you don't feel safe to or it's unfamiliar), you still feel that you have been forced. You oblige, but you do so with the same moodiness as a sullen teenager. You may keep the smile plastered on your face for fear of upsetting people, but inside you are furious.

If you feel resentful about having to do something, that's a good clue that it's violating a boundary of yours. Use that resentment as a signpost that there may be some self-abandonment going on here.

The resentment we feel with our partners is often coming from a childhood place. It's similar to the resentment we would have felt at being made responsible for other people or having our boundaries crossed when we were young. Still, no matter how resentful we feel at having to abandon our needs, we usually swallow this resentment (or it comes out in a passive-aggressive way), rather than actually saying no.

Why do we struggle to say no?

When we self-abandon, we choose a relationship over ourselves. Kelley's need to stay with Trish and her fear of abandonment may be so strong that she abandons her own needs and desires instead. The fact that she felt uncomfortable with sex 'being about her' gave me a clue that there might be some self-abandonment going on. Our survival-driven brain will do anything it can to prevent us being left, even if that means giving up on what we want. Essentially, we're abandoning ourselves so we don't get abandoned by our partner. This can be an attachment strategy – if we give our caregivers what we unconsciously sense they need, we don't get abandoned; we stay in the pack and don't get eaten by lions.

If you remember, Kelley and her mum are so close that her mum would talk to Kelley in detail about her sex life from a young age, and didn't like it when Kelley tried to have space. Kelley felt emotionally responsible for her mum (almost as though she was the parent), who was so sensitive to rejection that she couldn't bear it when Kelley was upset or tried to say no to things. This is what I'd think of as being an enmeshed mother–daughter relationship, where Kelley wasn't able to separate and become her own person. And now something similar is happening with Trish.

Generally, we struggle to set boundaries because we're afraid of the other person's response. Again, I think this comes back to the fear of abandonment because we fear being alone. If we grew up with a lack of boundaries, that might be how we experienced feeling close to someone else, in a merged way. So now we may equate boundaries and distance with feeling isolated and lonely.

I explore this with Kelley. She admits that if she says no to Trish, it will make her angry. 'Where did you first learn that it wasn't OK to say no?' I ask.

She thinks back. A memory of her mum bursting into tears. She's seven and she doesn't want to hug her mum. 'You don't love me any more, do you?' her mum says, tears streaming down her face. Kelley panics – a familiar anxiety; she doesn't want to make her mum upset. So, through gritted teeth, she forces herself to put her arms around her mum, who pulls her in so tightly it makes it hard to breathe. Kelley's body is rigid, but she knows she has to do this to make it better.

This is one small moment of many that would have happened during Kelley's childhood, telling her that she cannot have the space and independence she needs, undermining her boundaries and teaching her that she needs to abandon herself to make other people happy.

How do I heal?

Healing from co-dependency is absolutely possible. It takes both partners to really focus on healing themselves (and not the other person). So, how do you actually do this?

It involves the hard work of connecting to the wound and then taking action to enforce boundaries and meet your own needs. This can be painful (I know because I've done it, and continue to do it, myself). It requires going deep into your childhood, meeting your child self and really feeling what it was like to have your own needs pushed aside, to have to put others first, for your caregivers not to see or bear your feelings. It's not easy. It can feel like the most painful thing in the world at times, to be so vulnerable and hurt, but it is worthwhile. Processing the pain helps that wound to heal, so we don't recreate those wounds so much in our relationships.

Leaving the relationship might be helpful, but if you don't get to the root underneath you may just continue finding the same type of person and repeating this kind of relationship again.

As I said earlier, we heal through relationships with others. As Kelley starts to experiment with boundaries in our relationship, and expresses difference with me, she learns that it's safe and can start to apply this to her other relationships. I acknowledge that it's hard for her not to know anything about me, that there is a boundary between us, and I wonder if she's finding that uncomfortable. She nods. That separation is hard; she's not used to a relationship that is so separate. Acknowledging the feeling seems to help; she starts to come to sessions on time, asks fewer questions about me.

Therapy is a relationship where you can start to practise feeling or saying things that don't feel safe in your outside relationships. It's always a poignant moment when a patient who hasn't been able to express anger before tells me for the first time that they are angry with me. Or a patient who is highly independent and has always denied their need for others tells me, in a small, vulnerable voice, that they're afraid one day I might leave.

One of the main fears of changing is losing the relationship. While this can happen, it's not for certain. And at some point you have to ask yourself: are you willing to stay in a relationship if it comes at the cost of yourself?

This was the dilemma Kelley faced as she started to recognise the problem.

Five (non-exhaustive) things to help you heal from co-dependency

1. **Process the core wound.** The core wound is usually what's compelling you to seek out these dysfunctional patterns. Rather than blaming your partner, try to get in touch with what it is you're repeating. Were you made to feel controlled as a child, as though you couldn't say no? Or maybe you felt very out of control and needed to control others to feel safe? What was that like for you? Are there any memories or feelings you remember? Gently, get to know the hurt child in you who is replaying those wounds today.

2. **Get in touch with your intuition and needs**. It's important to notice your physical reaction when the urge to self-abandon comes up. When someone asks you to do something, what does your body say? Do you have a twinge of irritation and resentment, or does it feel calm and accepting? You don't necessarily have to respond differently yet, but just connect to your intuition to see whether your needs are in conflict with theirs. This is really about building trust in yourself again, so that little child inside you can trust that you'll be there for it after years of feeling abandoned.

3. **Take active steps to create healthy distance in your relationships.** As well as processing your childhood relationships, you also need to make changes in your adult relationships. Acknowledging and protecting your

difference is an important part of feeling whole. Healthy inter-dependence (where you depend on each other, but you can also mostly meet your own needs and look after yourself) requires a degree of separation. It's important to recognise that you are different people, with different feelings, desires, thoughts, values, likes and dislikes. This can be hard for many of us to tolerate, thinking we need to do all the same things as our partner, have all the same friends, like all the same places, agree on everything. Maintaining this healthy boundary between you stops you from making each other responsible for the other. Your partner is not responsible for your feelings, and you are not responsible for theirs. Celebrate your differences – that's probably what attracted them to you in the first place.

4. **Communicate.** A big part of separation is communication. Telling someone how you feel is in itself creating separation, because you're acknowledging that your feelings are not the same, that they can't read your mind. If you feel resentment building up, make sure you express your anger to your partner (in a measured and constructive way). When your anger is owned and expressed with compassion, rather than uncontained and taken out on the other person, it can be a helpful tool to create separation between you, because you are respecting yourself by saying that something is not OK with you. Self-respect is a barrier to co-dependency; because you're sticking up for yourself and meeting your own needs, you won't have to use others to meet those needs or abandon them entirely. The response

from others won't always be positive. You might not feel safe enough to express yourself in every relationship. In abusive adult relationships, it may indeed be the case that you will be punished for saying no. I understand that sometimes staying quiet and not causing a problem is a survival strategy. It's important that you check in with yourself about whether the relationship feels safe enough for you to speak up.

5. **Set boundaries.** Boundaries are the antidote to people-pleasing and co-dependency. They are how we distinguish between us and them. Setting a boundary draws a line between us and others, helping us separate our needs and feelings from theirs, and feel like a whole and strong person. Boundaries are protective. They are what we may not have had as children. They are an expression of difference: 'I do not want to do that. I have a separate mind from you. I can love you and be there for you and still want to do things differently.'

How to set boundaries

There are three key steps to setting boundaries:

1. **Identify what your boundary is.** Before you can set the boundary you need to be clear on exactly what you are and aren't prepared to put up with.

2. **Communicate.** Without blaming or attacking your partner, clearly state your boundary and the consequence if it's not respected.

3. **Enforce the boundary.** Boundaries need consequences, otherwise they're just empty words. Take action if your boundary is not respected, even if this makes the other person upset.

I'd encourage you to start small. We're trying to teach your mind that saying no is not the scary threat it thinks it is, so start with something manageable. Say no to a movie you don't want to watch, or to going to an event you're not fussed about. It will feel scary at first; you might experience a fear response (see page 52), but that isn't a reason to cave. Eventually, as your brain learns that boundaries are safe, you can progress to bigger and scarier boundaries.

Remember that boundaries are actions, not words. Most people don't realise that boundaries need to be acted on. If we don't enforce the boundary, then we are just teaching people that our words are meaningless and that there are no real consequences to their behaviour. For example, if you don't like the way someone speaks to you, you can ask them to speak differently, but if they don't do that then the boundary would be ending the conversation. The consequences allow us to control our boundaries rather than giving the power to someone else. If the person continues to violate your boundary and ignore the consequences then you might have to increase the consequences and, sad as it is, pull away from the relationship if nothing changes.

That being said, it is also important to bear in mind the other person. I often see an overcorrection when people start learning to express their feelings and needs. Because it can feel so frightening, people can become overly rigid or blame the other person. At the same time as expressing your needs, you have to find a way to negotiate and respect your partner's needs too. After all, no two people's needs will ever be 100 per cent the same, so it's such an important life skill to be able to both acknowledge and empathise with another's wants, and then explain calmly and compassionately why you need something different.

When I first started stating my boundaries, I found the whole thing so terrifying that I became a little selfish and aggressive in the way I was communicating. It was like a pendulum that swung too far. As someone from an enmeshed family myself, I used to often struggle to say no to events I didn't want to attend for fear that family members would think badly of me or that I'd let them down. There were three scenarios I moved through to get to what feels like a place of healthy communication:

1. **No communication.** Saying yes even when I wanted to say no, forcing myself to go to the event but finding it miserable and resenting the person for 'making me' go.

2. **Unhealthy communication.** Getting angry that they had dared to tell me I had to go to the event, shouting that they were manipulative and selfish, staying home in an angry huff and then feeling guilty that I'd been so unreasonable.

3. **Healthy communication.** Calmly explaining that I didn't want to go to the event, recognising that this was disappointing for them (and bearing their upset) and offering a compromise that met my need not to go, while also making them feel cared for.

Over time, after many failed attempts and boundaries that were too forceful, I was able to move to a place where I could communicate my needs while also considering the other person.

It all sounds fairly simple, but we all know too well that boundaries are harder to negotiate than they sound. Why? Because boundaries can upset other people, they can make people dislike us or feel angry with us, and this is something many of us struggle with. This is the challenge for any people pleaser: to tolerate not being liked. And people will not always react well to your boundaries, especially those who benefited from your lack of boundaries (and your family, who moulded you into being this way).

Remind yourself that you don't need everyone to like you at all times. It's OK if people are hurt or upset or mad – you will withstand it (even if your survival instincts are telling you otherwise). Their reaction is not your responsibility. It's usually less painful to live honestly and learn to accept that other people might not always like it.

What if you're the more controlling one?

Co-dependent relationships have two sides: the one who is demanding and controlling, and the one who is self-abandoning and lacks boundaries. I realise I'm speaking more to the side who struggle with self-abandonment and people-pleasing because that's what I tend towards, and it's also what I see more of in my practice. Still, we all have the capacity to be more like Trish – controlling and demanding, relying on our partners to save us, as if they were our parent.

However, there may be some of you reading this who, like Trish, want your partners to fit in with you and meet your needs. If you recognise yourself in Trish, it's so important to acknowledge this and not shame yourself for it – because that's the only way you'll be able to work on it. This, too, is likely coming from a childhood wound. Perhaps you experience a partner disagreeing with you as rejection and abandonment, like Kelley's mum. Maybe you're repeating what your parents were like with you. Or perhaps being demanding about getting your needs met makes you feel in control. It's just as important for you to trace back to the source of this pattern, and then try to learn in your adult relationships that a partner disagreeing or wanting to do something different doesn't mean that they don't love you.

What happens when someone changes in a relationship?

People might not always like it when you change.

'Something weird happened,' Kelley tells me. 'Trish told me to stop coming to therapy.'

Nursing a hangover, Trish took up her usual position in bed, crying into Kelley's arms. Kelley felt her fingers start to wring and remembered what we'd talked about, that she isn't responsible for people's feelings. 'Sorry you're feeling bad, babe,' she says, 'but I'm going to meet Dana to go to this exhibition.'

Trish flashed with panic. 'You can't leave me alone, I'm too depressed without you. Can you stay? I need you.' Kelley's fingers twisted, her knuckles turning white.

'I'm sorry you're having a hard time, but I can't fix this for you. I can't be your carer,' she says, her voice trembling.

'Is that something your therapist has told you to say?' Trish snaps, letting go of Kelley's hand.

'Well, yeah, actually, in a way. Therapy has made me realise how co-dependent we are, and that I'm not responsible for making you feel better.'

'I don't think therapy is helping, babe,' Trish replies, facing away. 'All she's doing is turning you against me.'

Kelley's holding her breath. She's stuck, caught between her old familiar way of being and the new self she's forming that can say no and puts herself first. She exhales and tells Trish as firmly as she can that she needs a bit of time to herself and she'll be back later.

When one partner changes it can disrupt the status quo. It's common for partners to feel threatened by therapy, because that's what is creating the change. *This is not a reason to stop changing*. If your partner likes the old, wounded version of you, ask yourself if this is a healthy place for you to develop and heal. Often we grow out of relationships as we heal, but this doesn't mean they all have to end. For this relationship to work, it seems that Trish needs to do some work on herself. If she does, perhaps the two of them can move into a more inter-dependent way of being.

Inter-dependence: the holy grail

Eventually, the aim is to move from co-dependence to inter-dependence. Inter-dependence is a more balanced, equal relationship, in which you feel like two separate people who are choosing to build a relationship together, rather than two half-people who cannot exist without the other.

There is nothing wrong with depending on someone – I think of this as being very healthy – but inter-dependence is about depending on them while still maintaining your sense of self. There's freedom within your committed and intimate relationship. You feel safe to rely on each other and turn to each other when you need to, and also safe to be yourself and have healthy distance. There may still be compromise when your needs are conflicting, but this is more balanced, like a seesaw going back and forth.

It's hard and the guilt snowballs, but Kelley keeps practising saying no, looking after her own needs and feeling whole outside of the relationship.

As Kelley begins to change, something miraculous starts to happen. Trish starts to get better.

Kelley first notices it on a night out. Usually, she closely monitors Trish's drinking, telling her when she's had enough and begging her to stop. This time, Kelley has vowed not to intervene. On Trish's third drink, when Kelley would normally be suggesting they switch to water, she says nothing. It's hard; she literally bites on her bottom lip to stop herself from saying anything, trying to breathe through the irritation of watching Trish order a fourth drink. Then, as someone orders another round, Trish yawns. 'I don't want to get too drunk actually. Shall we go home, babe?' Kelley is stunned. This has never happened before. For the first time, she realises that the more she treats Trish as a child, the more she becomes one. When Kelley stopped trying so hard to help her and act as the parent, Trish was able to moderate her own drinking and to parent herself.

When one person changes in a relationship, it often influences the other. While this might not always be for the best (partners resistant to change might do everything they can to sabotage the other's progress), sometimes it can shake up the dynamic in a positive way. With Kelley no longer acting as the parent, Trish moves out of the child role. This adult-to-adult relating is closer to the realm of inter-dependence, where each party looks after their own needs while still supporting the other.

A few weeks later, Kelley sits down, her hands resting calmly in her lap without fidgeting. I notice how much less anxious she seems. Something feels lighter.

'We had a big talk,' she says, exuding relief in her voice, 'and Trish is getting therapy.'

After a setback where Trish broke down and begged Kelley to cancel her plans to look after her, something in Kelley snapped. 'I don't think you realise how hard this is for me,' she said, crying. 'I can't look after you. It's draining me and making me so anxious, like you're this child I'm responsible for, like I can't have my own life without feeling like I'm letting you down. I love you but I can't save you, and I'll lose myself trying.'

'Were you saying that to Trish, or to your mum?' I ask.

She smiles at me. 'Both?'

While it was a hard conversation, Kelley's vulnerability shifted their dynamic once more. Instead of Kelley being the fixer and Trish the one in need, this time it was Kelley who was expressing some pain. This allowed Trish to be the one to care for Kelley this time. 'I didn't realise how this was all affecting you,' she said, taking Kelley into her arms. 'I'm so sorry – it's not fair to put all this on you.'

Later that night, Trish sat down next to Kelley. 'I've emailed this therapist. I don't want to burden you with my stuff any more. Seeing how you're changing is making me want to do the same.'

It takes time for them to rebalance their relationship, and they fall back into old patterns again and again. The difference is, they're both willing to reflect, learn and try to do things differently afterwards. And as Trish grows strong and more able, Kelley finds herself opening up in a more vulnerable way. She lets herself be the one to accept care and starts talking to Trish about some of the issues she's had with her mum. She's surprised at how willing and able Trish is to support her. As their relationship rebalances, they move towards inter-dependence, where each of them is looking after themselves, while still looking out for the other.

Signs of inter-dependence

- Having healthy boundaries.
- A sense of separateness.
- Showing up for each other.
- Taking responsibility for yourself and not blaming the other.
- Being vulnerable and open with each other.
- Communicating clearly, being able to express difference.

I'm aware that not all co-dependent relationships end like Kelley and Trish's – there will be many cases where leaving is the best option. However, we're often told to end a relationship as soon as these kinds of cracks start to appear, when actually change is possible, as long as both parties are committed to working on themselves.

FIGHTING AND COMMUNICATION

How Can I Stop Having the Same Fight with My Partner?

Giorgia and Dexter have been having the same fight for twenty years. The fight is about cleaning, except it has nothing to do with cleaning. It's usually Dexter who starts it.

Dexter gets home from a long day of work. Giorgia has left the kitchen in a state of disarray. His neck feels hot. Huffing and grunting, he tidies, grumbling to himself about how she has no respect, how this always happens. Once everything is clean, he passive-aggressively channels his annoyance into kneading a loaf of bread to demonstrate his care and make her feel guilty about her comparative negligence.

When they met at university, Giorgia was an international student visiting for the semester. Her messiness was part of her charm. She came to lectures in odd socks, papers falling out of her bag, with her long, thick hair knotted in a floppy bun. Dexter would gaze at her, wondering how to make her fall in love with him. He is quite the opposite, comfortable only in crisp white shirts and shiny shoes. They laughed at how different they were, 'like chalk *e formaggio*', she'd joke. Two kids, four moves and countless arguments later, Giorgia's messiness is no longer so appealing.

She comes home a ball of chaos, talking at a hundred miles an hour about a drama that happened at work. She dumps her bags in the hall, throws her shoes and socks on the floor, makes a cup of tea, leaving the spoon, milk AND teabag on the kitchen work surface, and slumps down on the sofa, all without mentioning the newly cleaned kitchen or the smell of bread in the oven.

Dexter is ready to blow. He tells her she's inconsiderate, that she's a slob and a princess who expects everyone else to pick up after her. His neck grows redder. She doesn't think about anyone but herself. Selfish, that's what Giorgia is.

Giorgia is exhausted. Her boss has been breathing down her neck all day and made her stay late, again. She spent every minute watching the clock waiting for the moment when she could take off her shoes and chill on the sofa with a cup of tea. Dexter is still shouting. She slams down the mug, abandoning any hope of a relaxing evening, and shouts back. Can't he lay off her for a second? Why does he have to be so anal and controlling? Can't he see that she's stressed and doesn't need any more on her plate? He's the selfish one.

Dexter's neck turns a shade redder. He brings up the time Giorgia was an hour late to the movie he'd got tickets for and he had to watch the first half alone. She brings up the time he had a go at her for cutting bread the wrong way. Soon they forget what they were arguing about in the first place.

Bread. 'Oh no,' Dexter says, his eyes widening as he realises.

'Is that burning?' Giorgia asks.

Smoke streams from the oven as Dexter removes the black ball of coal he spent so long meticulously kneading. He's fuming now, his neck practically purple. He screams that this is all Giorgia's fault, that it's like living with a child. She clearly doesn't care about him at all. She calls him a control freak and a narcissist. 'You sound just like your mother,' she snaps.

He throws the bread in the bin and storms upstairs. Her tea grey and cold, Giorgia is left on the sofa wondering how they ended up having this same fight yet again.

The content of the fight is often not the real reason you're fighting. It's the tip of the iceberg. What's underneath is usually something that has threatened your attachment relationships. So what *were* Dexter and Giorgia arguing about?

Dexter experienced Giorgia's mess as a rejection of him. She didn't tidy because she took him for granted. When she came home without recognising his efforts, and messed them up again, Dexter felt even more disrespected. This may have triggered something from his past. His mum could be critical, always nitpicking and making him feel like he was doing things wrong. He used to try to impress her by finishing all his homework, tidying his bedroom and being good. Except she never noticed. She'd come home, ignore the efforts he'd put in and tell him off for looking scruffy or not putting away his bag. Unbeknown to Dexter, when Giorgia doesn't acknowledge the clean kitchen, those same feelings of being ignored and criticised come careering back. His reaction is coming from the little boy inside him who never felt like he was enough. Of course, some of you might have realised – just as Giorgia did – that Dexter has become controlling and critical, just like his mum. I would guess that somewhere along the intergenerational chain, Dexter's mum was also made to feel rejected and controlled, and so the cycle is being repeated.

We internalise our parents and, despite desperately wanting to be nothing like them, often end up repeating the exact things we wish they hadn't done. Of course, some of us try to rebel and swing towards the exact opposite way of being, but often we can't avoid taking on the traits of our parents.

One of the reasons for this is because we haven't learnt another way to communicate. Dexter's mum never taught him to share his feelings, and instead he learned to express hurt by being critical of others. So now, when Dexter is feeling rejected by Giorgia, he doesn't know how to communicate that. All he knows is criticism and control.

– EXERCISE –

Reflect on the type of arguments you tend to have with people, if any. Are you honestly communicating how you feel? Are you fighting about something seemingly unrelated, like Dexter and Giorgia? Are you conflict averse, or passive-aggressive, indirectly communicating your anger?

Now think about how this maps onto your family's way of fighting – what was modelled to you as a child? Can you remember a specific fight you witnessed or were aware of as a child? If you can't remember any fighting at all, that's interesting to note too.

What kind of communication style does your family have? How did your parents or siblings argue, if they argued at all? And what was the frequency of the arguments? Was there lots of fighting, did nothing get talked about or were you taught how to talk openly about what was upsetting you? How might this link to how you tend to fight now?

How do we communicate differently?

Vulnerability is the antidote here. Rather than retaliating, try to connect to the feelings that have been triggered and express them to your partner. If you can find a way to communicate that you're hurt, you can start to have a more healing kind of conversation.

The first step is awareness. Dexter has to recognise that he's hurt before he can change his approach. When you start feeling annoyed with someone, blaming them, wanting to shout or make passive-aggressive comments or hurt them in some way, this is a sign that something has been triggered in you. Before reacting, take a moment to connect with what's hurting. By reflecting on what's going on under the surface, Dexter comes to realise that his anger might be about something more than just the mess.

Let's play the situation again to see how they could respond differently.

The next time Giorgia leaves the house a mess and Dexter resentfully tidies it, he notices his neck get hot again. He's been ranting at her in his head all afternoon, waiting for her to come home so he can shout. Then he stops. Noticing all the pent-up frustration in his body, he takes a moment to regulate his nervous system. He lies on the bed upstairs and takes ten deep breaths. Things feel a little better; the anger simmers down.

This moment of awareness is key – it stops Dexter from being so reactive. 'Get curious,' he remembers hearing. He takes a moment. 'What am I feeling?' he asks himself. 'I'm feeling rejected,' a voice replies, 'like you don't care, like you're ignoring my hard work just like my mum used to.' He thinks about that little boy inside him, sad and unloved. The anger creeps back up, but, sick of the same argument, he knows he doesn't want to take it out on Giorgia.

By understanding and sitting with the hurt that has been triggered, Dexter is able to put some distance between him and his reactive anger. He waits for Giorgia to get home, take off her shoes and enjoy her cup of tea. His neck is still red, but he breathes through it. Then, when he's finished listening to Giorgia's stressful day, he tries a different approach.

He starts with 'I feel'. 'I feel hurt when you leave all the tidying to me. Mess makes me stressed, and I know you know that, so when you leave things messy it feels like you don't care about me and aren't thinking about me. Then, when you don't notice me cleaning up after you, I feel rejected all over again. I know it's silly,' he says, 'but it really does hurt me. It triggers some stuff with my mum that makes me feel like a little boy again who no one cares about. It makes me really angry, but I don't want to be controlling like her.'

Giorgia, sensing how difficult this is for Dexter to say, puts her arm round him. 'I'm sorry, babe,' she says, 'I didn't realise that. I can be chaotic. I know that's not fun – I just don't love being told what to do, so sometimes I rebel against you like you're a parent or something. But I thought you were just nagging for no reason. I didn't realise it was because it was making you feel like I didn't care.' She kisses his head. 'Of course I care about you. I'll try to make more of an effort to show you that.'

Dexter takes the bread out of the oven, and they enjoy slices of thick buttery toast together on the sofa.

Because Dexter led with his feelings, rather than criticising Giorgia's character, Giorgia doesn't need to jump on the defence. She can empathise with him and reflect on her own behaviour because she doesn't feel so attacked. By owning and expressing his vulnerability, Dexter has done something incredibly brave and introduced a new way of communicating – one where he shares his hurt, rather than trying to retaliate and hurt back. By staying with their own feelings, rather than attacking each other, they can put their weapons down and meet each other from a loving place.

Rupture and repair is key to healing

Rupture and repair is something we talk about a lot in therapy. Ruptures occur in all relationships, but it's how we repair those ruptures that affects the relationship and our own emotional wellbeing. The ruptures might look similar to the ones you had in childhood, or the kind of arguments and tensions your parents modelled. Healing is about repairing these ruptures in a way that's different from how they were dealt with in childhood, so you can learn new, healthier ways of handling conflict. It's through repairing these ruptures that we can come out stronger, more connected and better understood.

NB This might not be the case for relationships that are abusive. You need to make sure you only express your hurt and vulnerability to a person with whom you feel safe, who will hold it with the care and tenderness it deserves (of course, none of us is perfect – sometimes we don't respond to our loved ones from a place of care and tenderness – but it should be someone you think will generally respond with care). If you're reading this and feel worried that you might be in an abusive relationship, I'd encourage you to talk to a person you can trust – a friend, family member or professional. There are services and helplines in the back of this book if you need support (see page 317).

How to have difficult conversations

Here are a few of my golden rules for communication. They might take a while to master – it's all about trial and error.

- **Stick to 'I feel' statements.** When you start by putting the blame on someone else, they can immediately feel attacked and go into defensive mode. Take accountability for your own feelings, rather than listing all the things they've done wrong. Take the heat off and just tell them how their actions make you feel, e.g. 'I feel hurt when you . . .' is much less attacking than, 'You did this and it hurt me . . .'

- **Think about what you might be projecting onto them**. Are they really being critical, or are you projecting your own criticisms onto them? Was Giorgia really doing anything wrong by being messy, or was Dexter projecting his insecurities onto her? Before you launch into blaming someone else, try to reflect on how much is your own stuff and what you can take accountability for.

- **Acknowledge their feelings.** Research shows that conflict is lessened in couples if they can understand each other's feelings and perspectives. Even if you don't agree, acknowledging how they're feeling and letting them know that you care about their perspective can go a long way.

- **Try to tolerate the discomfort of the fear of not being liked or making someone angry.** If you're conflict averse, difficult conversations can feel very frightening. To really say what you think and communicate openly, you have to learn not to look after the other person's feelings so much. If you're a people pleaser it can be hard to be assertive, which is why it takes practise. Remind yourself that it's not your job to keep them happy, and avoiding topics that might upset someone is a form of self-abandonment. By avoiding conflict, you're prioritising their needs (or at least the needs you're imagining they have) over your own.

- **Try to communicate when regulated.** The rule that you should never go to bed during a fight is a myth, in my opinion. Having conversations when one or both of you are dysregulated is usually unhelpful – things tend to escalate without each of you really hearing the other because you're too busy reacting. Sometimes, the more avoidant person might need to withdraw in order to regulate their emotions – and that's OK. Don't be afraid to take breaks. Pause, go into separate rooms, breathe. Then, once both of you feel calm again, approach the conversation from a more regulated, less defensive place. Of course, we're all human – it might not always be possible for both people to regulate themselves before talking. Sometimes one might need to apologise, especially if one has said something particularly hurtful; sometimes one will need to 'go first' to help the other regulate. What's also important is that after the apologies, when you've both calmed a little, there is real communication and mutual understanding of what happened.

- **Be curious and listen.** When we raise an issue, sometimes we can be focused on getting out everything we want to say, rather than listening to the other person. It's so important that both people really take the time to listen to each other and empathise as best they can, rather than jumping to the defence or attack. Even when the conversation is hard it can be mutually supportive if you respect the other's point of view and expect them to respect yours.

'It's easier to be different with new people.' This is something my therapist says to me often. What she means (I think) is that it's very hard to start acting differently with people who are used to us acting in a certain way. It's much easier to set boundaries and communicate with people we've just met, because they don't know us as the boundary-lacking, poor communicators we once were.

Society values old relationships. We romanticise high school sweethearts and feel we need to stay close with the people we went to school with. Even if we've become radically different people who no longer get on, we cling on to old friendships because they are valued as superior. In reality, it can be easier to make changes in new friendships, because they're meeting you as you are now, changes already in place.

It's not one-size-fits-all, of course. Profound healing can also take place within your old relationships, especially if you're able to change as a whole, such as in family therapy, where you heal together. It can be helpful to practise being different with someone new in your life first, and work up to implementing these new ways of being with the people already in your life.

Section Four
Out of the Relationship

CHEATING

Why Do People Cheat?

Maeve comes to see me without passion or desire. She seems quite nervous, as most people are in the first session, clutching her bag on her lap and not taking off her grey pea coat. 'Are you going to record this?' she asks, suspicious. I take this to mean that she doesn't quite trust me – and why should she? I'm a stranger at this point – I assure her that this is entirely confidential, and nothing will be recorded.

She puts her bag down. We begin.

Maeve has recently gone back to work as a solicitor after having her second child, and she's struggling to get her sense of identity back. Everything feels dull and meaningless. At work she feels incapable because she's distracted thinking about the kids, and at home she feels like a failure for not being far enough along in her career. It's a lot to handle on her own; I ask how her partner helps to support her. 'I don't want to come to therapy to talk about Finn,' she says. I register the defensive response and let her continue.

Minutes later, she's telling me about a meltdown she had when Finn gave the kids sugar before bed and they were chasing each other round the kitchen while she was trying to work on some–

Her lips seal shut mid-sentence. 'I don't want to talk about him,' she says again.

'It's you who brought him up,' I say playfully. She doesn't laugh or even crack a smile. There's something uptight about her that makes it hard for me to connect.

In not talking about Finn, there seems to be something she's keeping out, something she doesn't want to confront or put words to. I try to be patient and let the story come out in its own time.

The next session, she puts her bag on the floor and unbuttons her coat, though she still keeps it on. She mentions Finn in a small and safe way, a minor complaint about how he works late, leaving her to look after the kids on her own. Again, I make a mental note of this but decide not to scare her away by asking too many questions too early. She makes a joke about how it's like having three kids, not two. As she shares more, the resentment starts to seep out of the lips she's trying to keep shut. By the fourth session, the grievances roll in thick and fast. Finn works too much. When he's home he's too tired to engage with her or help much. She's left to tidy the house, sort the kids' food, get them to bed, all while trying to balance her own career too. Meanwhile Finn sits on the sofa, watching football or going off to the pub with his friends.

In our sixth session, Maeve comes back in with her coat fully buttoned and clutching her bag once again. She tells me it's a relief to talk about Finn; she's been too afraid that talking about it will make it worse, but it's good to get it off her chest. Her words don't quite square with her body language – her bag is quite literally blocking the chest she's telling me is now free. It's like she needs the coat and the bag to hold something in once again. What else is she keeping close to her chest?

'The thing about Finn,' she continues, 'is that he was mollycoddled by his mum. He had everything handed to him on a silver platter, and now he expects me to do the same.'

'Have you ever spoken to him about this,' I ask?

'No,' she says.

'So what are you doing about it?'

Maeve's head bows, her eyes darting from side to side as if she's deciding her next move. It's a look of panic and shame, one that's telling me to go gently. So I don't push, and wait for her to speak.

She sighs deeply, resolved to tell me.

Joe is a man from work she has been flirting with. It was harmless at first, a few jokes by the coffee machine, lingering eye contact in team meetings, silly texts. Then, one night after work drinks, they found themselves alone after everyone had left. His fingers brushed hers as he told her boldly that she was beautiful. Maeve felt more alive than she had in years.

When she tells me about the affair now, she is full of guilt and regret, yet there's an excitement in her voice. The charge is palpable; I can feel it between us as she tells me how they would have sneaky kisses in the office kitchen and linger at the end of socials so they could be alone again. She knows it's wrong; a part of her feels terrible, but another part needs this affair to feel alive. I find myself getting drawn in, almost revelling in the excitement of it all. Suddenly Maeve has gone from being a patient I couldn't quite connect with to someone thrilling and intriguing. I wonder if this is how Maeve feels about herself.

'You're enjoying this,' I say. Maeve looks down sheepishly. 'You're a different person when you talk about the affair – it's like you've come to life.'

Maeve nods. 'I know, it's terrible. I feel like a teenager again, like someone who's mysterious and interesting. Then I think of Finn and the girls and I feel like the worst mother who's ever existed. If they found out – God, I don't know what I'd do. But every time I try to stop, I can't. He's like a drug that's the only thing making me feel something.'

Now, some of you might be judging Maeve, might agree that she's a terrible mother, that she should feel ashamed, but that is not my job. As I sit with her, I'm trying to understand why – why does Maeve need to cheat? What function is it serving for her? Is the affair making her feel desired, creating a sense of mystery and excitement? Is she furious with Finn and enacting her anger through the affair? Or is she self-sabotaging, ruining her family life because a part of her doesn't believe she deserves it, or because she's used to a more chaotic and broken family? I don't know the reason, and of course there might be many, but this is for us to uncover together.

Reasons for infidelity

There are different types of cheating and different reasons for cheating. Many people don't have a sense of the reason why they cheat – if you ask them, they'll say they don't know. That doesn't mean there isn't a reason, just that the reason is unconscious. I'm aware that not all affairs are like Maeve's, one-off and guilt-ridden. There are people who cheat chronically; 'fuckboys' who get off on messing people around; people who cheat out of pressure from friends and laugh about it with them; people who fall in love with someone else and keep the affair hidden for years; people who self-sabotage by spoiling something good; people who need a secret; people who cheat out of revenge or anger, or who love their partner but have stopped wanting to have sex with them.

While I'm focusing on monogamous relationships here, cheating can still take place within non-monogamous relationships. When someone crosses a boundary that is defined within the relationship it can still be a transgression.

Many believe cheating comes from pure cruelty, but actually it can come from something deeper. People often cheat not just because of sex, but to escape. Relationships are riddled with conflict and reveal our deepest wounds and insecurities. Cheating allows people to escape into a fantasy where conflict doesn't exist, where the other person is perfect. They're running away from the person intimacy has revealed them to be. Take Jay, who would desperately search for a relationship and then end up cheating on the women he fell for. This is the kind of cheating that protects people against intimacy. By ruining the relationship and hurting people in the process, they never have to risk actually getting close to someone.

Often, it's about feeling either too close and needing distance (like Maeve) or not close enough and needing connection elsewhere, or fearing closeness altogether (like Jay). Most people don't cheat because they're evil; they cheat because they're hurting or craving something different.

Now, I'm obviously not condoning cheating – it can cause a lot of hurt for a lot of people. If there was an expectation of the relationship that was violated, that's not OK. If you've been cheated on, you get to decide if that's a hurt that you can recover from.

The cheater is not innocent – they crossed a boundary, which is hurtful, but it's nuanced. While it might make us feel a little better in the moment to demonise cheating and categorise cheaters as evil people with no moral compass, it's only going to make the problem harder to discuss as it becomes shrouded in shame.

Whatever the reason, my understanding is that cheating is a way of acting out and communicating what cannot be spoken. So if we can openly and vulnerably talk to each other about how we feel, we're less likely to act upon these feelings by being unfaithful.

In most of the examples above, if the cheater could talk about their shameful or difficult feelings with their partner, they might not need to act upon them. When we feel as though we can't talk to our partners about how we feel, afraid of hurting them or making them angry, those feelings (whether it's fear, anger, feeling unwanted, longing for something different or even being attracted to someone else) are acted upon instead of worked through.

Maeve

I don't do much. It isn't about tools or homework or giving Maeve anything to DO; the therapy here is about providing her with a place to discuss her fears without being shamed. Shame and fear are two of the reasons Maeve hasn't been able to talk to Finn about what's missing in their relationship, and so those feelings have been acted upon in her seeking out Joe. To lessen the shame, I want to do everything I can to make it OK for Maeve to say whatever she wants here without feeling judged. That being said, it's important I don't exempt her from any responsibility either. I don't want to walk her away from her own sense of morality. Still, these situations aren't straightforward. She's caused great hurt in having this affair, but she's also hurting herself.

It's not easy to own up to your mistakes and confront the ways you're hurting others, which is why I believe it's so important to talk about our shadow sides to stop them from being acted upon. So often, cheating is an enactment of feelings that can't be spoken about. By giving Maeve a place where she can speak about these things, it might be that her need to act upon these feelings lessens.

One of the main problems, Maeve explains, is that she and Finn stopped having sex after the second baby came. It's not just because they were too tired and busy, but because she actively didn't want to go near him. When he'd try to cuddle up to her or kiss her before they went to sleep, her whole body would recoil in repulsion. It took every fibre of her being not to push him off her. Somewhere along the way she stopped seeing Finn as a sexual being.

Then, when Joe came along, he was so uncomplicated and undemanding. She didn't have to make him dinner or tidy up after him. Joe was a man, not another baby who needed looking after. There was something about Joe's manliness and independence that reawakened a part in Maeve she didn't know she'd lost – the part that wants to be seen as an adult, not as a mother.

Why don't I want to have sex with my partner any more?

One of the most common reasons for affairs is because the spark has gone, so people look elsewhere to be desired. They might deeply love their partners and want to be together, but their sexual needs are not being met by the relationship. In psychotherapist Esther Perel's book *Mating in Captivity*,[17] she noticed that it was so common for people to become less attracted to their long-term partners because being TOO close can extinguish desire.

Her theory is that when people are too close they start to feel like family. We want to feel close and be able to depend on our partners. We show our messy and vulnerable sides, share responsibilities, finances, children. They see us when we're sick and messy and at our worst. While this might make for a healthy relationship, it can also jeopardise mystery and passion. Our biological instincts are not to sleep with our family, so we don't feel attracted to them.

In a relationship there are two competing needs: safety and desire. We have to balance the need for closeness and familiarity with the need for attraction. If there's too much closeness, we might be less attracted to them as they feel too much like family. If there's too much distance and not enough safety, the chemistry might be great, but the emotional relationship won't be.

Reconnecting is about rebalancing these conflicting needs for safety and desire. If you're struggling with this, I'd encourage you to create some space in the relationship – maybe find separate hobbies or prioritise friends. Desire is about experiencing your partner as separate, as their own person.

A little distance creates a sense of mystery and playfulness, so you can remember what attracted you in the first place and come back together and reconnect. It's a cliché but going on date nights can really help you to see your partner as a romantic lover rather than just a co-parent, housemate or friend.

The problem with parent–child dynamics

Maintaining desire is especially hard in co-dependent relationships, or when one person feels like a carer for the other. We all have the ability to slip into parent or child mode – especially in close romantic relationships, as they are the most similar to our intimate family relationships.

Being in parent mode might look like being very nurturing and caring, but also critical and controlling, depending on the type of parenting you were exposed to. A partner with a strong parent state might enable the other person to occupy the child state, becoming helpless and passive and lacking in responsibility.

Many will unconsciously seek out a mummy or daddy in their adult partnerships, which, to some extent, works. They might find a partner who does everything for them, prioritises them, soothes them when they're in need. That is, until their partner starts to see them as a needy child and stops feeling attracted to them. They might have all their safety and care needs met, but it comes at the cost of attraction and desire.

Let's face it, it's not hot to look after someone who can't look after themselves. Of course, at times it's natural to slip into a parent role with our partners, when they're sick and need looking after or when they're going through a particularly stressful period, but if you're acting as the parent the majority of the time, it starts to get pretty unsexy to have an adult baby as a partner. The typical example is a 'man child', incapable of cooking or cleaning or doing anything for themselves while their wife waits on them hand and foot. It's unsurprising that she might not want to have sex with him any more, because she no longer sees him as an adult in a reciprocal relationship; instead, he is her son, needy and incapable. This is not a dynamic that is necessarily gendered – you also see men who bend over backwards to accommodate their female partners, feeling equally parentified.

If being in a parent role resonates with you, it's important to understand what it is you're getting from this dynamic. While you might feel resentful and bitter, I'm guessing there is a reason why you take up this role:

- Maybe you were made to act as the parent sometimes as a child, so it feels familiar.
- Maybe you struggle with boundaries and saying no, so you end up prioritising other people's needs over your own.
- Maybe being the carer makes you feel more secure in the relationship, because they're less likely to leave if they need you.
- Maybe you're projecting all your neediness and vulnerability onto them, so you can feel independent and strong.

Transactional Analysis

Transactional analysis, a type of psychotherapy founded by Eric Bern in the 1950s, believes we all have three states: the child, the parent and the adult[18]). The parent is us behaving like our parent figures, the child state brings back feelings and behaviours from when we were a child, and the adult is us behaving with awareness and control in the present. The state we are in depends on how we were parented in childhood, traumas that have conditioned us to act a certain way, and how the other person is acting. If someone is acting in child mode, that might trigger us to slip into parent mode.

The goal of transactional analysis is to help people stay in adult state, by noticing when they've slipped into a parent or child state. It's usually an unconscious way of being, so it's important that we are aware of when we've slipped into child or parent mode so we can come back to our adult way of relating.

If being more in the child role resonates with you, there will also be reasons (possibly unconscious), why you tend towards this state:

- Maybe you feel helpless and unable to do things for yourself. Perhaps your parents didn't nurture your sense of power and agency.
- Maybe you faced trauma at a young age, which is easily triggered, making you respond from a child place.
- Perhaps, because of early unmet needs, you feel others should look after you to make up for what you didn't get.
- Maybe you were forced to grow up too fast, so the child in you remains stuck and not emotionally developed.
- Perhaps there's something threatening about being in a stronger, less passive position.

These roles are mutually influential; the dynamic is between you and exacerbated by the other person (i.e. if we act like a child, we evoke the parent in the other, and vice versa). For example, Giorgia's messiness evokes Dexter's angry parent; Connor's avoidance triggers Abby's 'needy' child; Trish's drinking and helplessness brings out Kelley's over-responsible parent.

Maeve

Six months in, Maeve comes in and takes her coat off for the first time.

'I'm ready,' she says.

'Ready for what?'

She hangs her coat on the hook. 'To tell Finn.'

Over the last few months, as she's learnt to express her frustration and anger towards Finn, a whole bunch of other feelings have been given a voice too. Love, guilt, loneliness, anger at herself and fear for what will happen to their family when he finds out.

Keeping silent about the issues in the relationship is part of the reason she ended up having the affair. 'It'll be like dropping a bomb,' she explains, 'but at least it's an honest bomb, and maybe we can see what we can salvage from the wreckage.' It's not that she wants to break up – quite the opposite. She wants to tell him so they can rebuild into something new. There's hope in telling him, hope that he'll forgive her, hope that she can learn to communicate when she feels unsupported and too much like his parent. She's dropping the bomb in the hope that together they can create a different kind of relationship, one of equality and respect and desire.

'Wish me luck,' she says as she stands, fear wavering in her voice. She looks at me, eyes wide and determined. 'I know it's weird, but I'm kind of proud of myself.' I smile. I'm proud of her too. She takes her coat off the hook, buttons it up and leaves.

Why do I struggle to trust people?

People's sense of trust in others is based on their experience with their parents. If you didn't develop a sense of basic trust in your parents, cheating will bring up all of those wounds from childhood.

Babies enter the world as entirely trusting, because they have to be. If a child is loved and cared for well enough, they'll develop a sense of security and trust in others. Those with a secure attachment are more trusting than people who are insecurely attached. If a child has parents who are depressed, anxious, dismissive, too needy or angry, however, their ability to trust others may be damaged. If your parents weren't able to meet all your emotional needs, you might walk around with the blueprint that 'people let me down'. To protect ourselves, we build a system of defences to stop us being hurt again. We might promise not to trust people again, avoid relationships altogether, be vigilant for signs of betrayal and then feel vindicated when we spot them.

This blueprint might affect the type of partner you choose, making you more likely to choose unfaithful people and thereby creating a self-fulfilling prophecy when someone does cheat on or abandon you. You might think of yourself as someone very trusting, who just keeps choosing people who are deceitful, but in blindly ignoring red flags and focusing only on the good things, there may be an unconscious, wounded part of you that is choosing someone to repeat those childhood wounds of betrayal and mistrust in order to confirm what you've already experienced – that they will hurt you like everyone else has.

The more relationships we have where the trust is broken, the more our lack of trust snowballs. When your trust is repeatedly violated, your expectations of a relationship are likely to be negative. Once you've been cheated on once, you might be convinced that it'll happen with everyone else. It all stems from the original wound of being let down by the very people we relied upon to keep us safe, and then being hurt by the people who are supposed to love us.

How to rebuild trust when someone cheats

Learning to trust people is less about finding someone who will never hurt you, and more about learning to trust that you'll be able to handle it if they do.

- **Turn inwards rather than outwards.** You might feel very angry and want to lash out, but this likely isn't going to help you process what's happened. Of course your anger is valid and should be expressed, but try to focus on yourself rather than them. Give yourself some time to process the shock and hurt you're going through.

- **Reflect on the relationship.** Even though it's hard, be curious about your partner's reasons for cheating and be honest about your part in the difficulties in the relationship. Sometimes the cheater may be the one acting out, signalling that the relationship is in trouble and needs attention (though not always). This is not to take away from the hurt and anger, but to allow you to reflect on what went wrong.

- **Decide whether you want to stay or go.** Cheating is a deal breaker for many, but it doesn't always have to be the end of a relationship. If you think trust can be restored and the other person is willing and committed to working on what's gone wrong, there's no shame in trying. If you're thinking of staying, it's important to be aware of how the other person responds to the issues or conflict – are they defensive and unempathetic, or are they open and loving? If it's the former, the cheating might give you clarity that the relationship isn't right for you.

- **Communicate rather than act.** You might never want to speak to your partner again, and that is valid. Communication is still necessary, though, if you want to find a way to trust someone new. Being clear about how you've been hurt in the past and any fears you have is important, whether it's with the old or new partner, because this stops our trust issues from being acted out. Trust issues often push people away, and even become a self-fulfilling prophecy, when they aren't properly expressed. We only resort to controlling behaviours, such as going through their phone or dictating who they see, when we are afraid and mistrustful. If we can own and communicate that, we are far less likely to act upon it. By changing the way you communicate with each other, you might be able to find a way to trust again.

BREAK-UPS AND GRIEF

How Do I Get Over Someone?

It's two years since Maeve's divorce. She is still, understandably, struggling. She can't focus at work. She sits in the pub with friends tuning out. Her body is there, but she is dead inside. The only time she comes alive is when talking about Finn.

She comes in each week with a mania in her eyes, calculating schemes about how to get him to forgive her for the affair. Finn has made it clear: there is no going back. Still, she feeds off tiny details. A friend who saw him in a café looking sad, or a confused string of emojis at the end of a message about lawyers. When their son goes to stay with Finn at weekends, Maeve grills him and lives off the details for months.

Life moves on around her, friends move away, her sister falls pregnant, the team at work is restructured, but Maeve stays frozen. She cannot move forward, and she is miserable in her inertia.

Why is losing someone so hard?

It's normal to feel a range of emotions after a break-up (or any form of grief): fear, anger, sadness, shock, loneliness. It's a kind of death of the relationship, of your world as you know it, of your plans and hopes for the future.

When faced with loss it's healthy to feel the pain. By spending all day in your pyjamas, cancelling on friends, crying in the office loos, screaming down the phone to your mum, there is a kind of acceptance, an understanding that you have lost this person. Though it can feel heartbreaking, eventually the pain morphs into something more positive and productive, and this sense of progress allows you to move on and rebuild your world, even if the world looks different without that person.

This is what I'd consider a healthy kind of mourning. It might take longer than you'd like and it might be terribly painful, but it does shift and you can eventually move on.

Maeve is going through what I think of as a more complicated type of mourning, one she isn't moving on from, which is keeping her stuck. While normal grief shifts over time, with complicated grief the person struggles to get past it; they stay stuck in mourning, which stops them from being able to function properly.

In a complicated mourning, the loss might have triggered something that isn't bearable, so it gets stuck in the unconscious. Though Maeve is very much in pain, her stuckness says to me that there are feelings she isn't processing. Avoiding the grieving process stops us from having to accept it, which keeps us trapped in the past.

If you're struggling to get over someone, the loss might have become less about them and more about what you've lost from yourself. We lose parts of ourselves when we lose people, whether it's a romantic relationship, a friendship or someone who has died. We don't feel whole without them. Trying to get them back or still pining over them is part of the fantasy that you'll feel whole if you have them again.

Loss can make us question who we are without that person and leave us feeling as though we can't move forward on our own. This can prevent you from being open to someone new, making things feel even more stuck.

On a personal note, break-ups have usually broken me, and they've also provided a lot of growth and awareness about myself and what I want. If you avoid the grief, by clinging on to the person or numbing your feelings with alcohol, food and constant distraction, such as rebound relationships, the grief might be harder to let go of, making it harder to feel whole again in their absence. There are also other kinds of relationship endings that trigger grief. The ending of friendships is something that's not really spoken about, yet in my experience it brings up all the same feelings of abandonment and loss and low self-worth that a romantic break-up does.

Friendship break-ups

I still have nightmares about a particularly difficult friendship break-up. For years I was close with this person; we told each other all our secrets, went on holidays, called each other when we were walking somewhere late at night. She threw a surprise party for me when I finished my PhD, remembered the exact chocolate bar I liked when I was stressed and could recount my dating horror stories to our mutual friends better than I could. I naively assumed she'd be in my life forever. Then one day she ghosted me, for reasons I still don't understand. That was it. Someone who I considered a best friend was just out of my life, with no indication of why.

We didn't fall out, we didn't drift apart; she just stopped being my friend. The grief was intense and complicated.

My desperation was similar to the feeling of being dumped, except more confused because there was no dumping to speak of, just an absence. There was something about the lack of understanding that made it hard to process. I talked to mutual friends, stalked her Instagram, re-read our texts for clues of what went wrong. I have my theories – you've probably realised by now that I like to overanalyse things, which is useful for therapy, though not so useful for daily life – but I'll never really know.

At first, I judged myself for caring so much. Why was I feeling so devastated? Then I realised that this loss was just as painful as any other, that I needed to let myself grieve just as I would for a romantic relationship. You've lost an important person – it's OK to feel however you feel about this. Give those feelings space to be processed without judgement.

How do you grieve for a relationship?

If loss is something you're struggling with at the moment, first of all, I'm sorry. It's one of the most painful experiences you can go through, and there is no real remedy for that. Second, I hate to be the bearer of bad news, but the healthiest thing you can do is to go through it. The more you avoid it, the less able you'll be to really let go.

Have you allowed yourself to grieve? Really grieve? If not, why? Are you putting pressure on yourself to move on or get over it? What happens if you just let yourself feel exactly how you're feeling? Are you in denial about your pain? What would happen if you let it hurt just as much as it needs to?

Friendships

As you grow and change over the course of your life, you might naturally drift from some people. This doesn't make you a failure – you don't have to cling on to people who no longer fit you. Isn't it interesting, though, that many of us are prepared to put so much work into our romantic relationships – talking about how we feel, expressing our love, thinking carefully about the dynamics at play, even seeking couples therapy – yet when it comes to our friendships, we expect them to tick along nicely without putting in any work? All the dynamics I talk about in romantic relationships also exist in friendships. But because we don't tend to communicate with our friends in the same way as we do with romantic partners, many friendships stay stuck or break down.

Friendships are just as much a place to grow as romantic relationships. While it's perfectly normal to outgrow friendships, I wonder how many could be saved if we were able to talk about difficult things, rather than just pulling away when the going gets tough.

Phases of Grief

Many people go through five Elisabeth Kübler-Ross[19] stages of grief – denial, anger, bargaining, depression and acceptance. This might look different for everyone; we don't all necessarily go through the stages in order, and often people get stuck at a certain stage. This happens when we aren't accepting the loss because we're avoiding the very painful feelings that come with it. Maeve for example, is stuck in the denial and bargaining phases; she needs to move through the depression by processing the loss to come out the other side into acceptance and hope.

Grief is never fully 'completed', because it's something that we learn to live with. That said, it won't hurt as badly forever. It will be more complicated however, if you don't let it hurt at all. Let yourself feel every drop, so you can move forward and rebuild.

— *EXERCISE* —

Think of the main things you feel you've lost after the relationship. It can be anything: companionship, your shared friends, someone to go to events with, someone to make you feel loved. For each thing you've lost, name three ways you can fill that hole for yourself. Maybe you can ask your friends to go to those events with you, or spend time with family or friends who make you feel loved. Of course, there are some things we cannot replace, and for those we will have to let ourselves feel the pain of that loss, but this might also be an opportunity to make changes in our life that help us feel whole again.

Now think of three things you lost during the relationship. Did you lose closeness with certain people, give up things you like to do, have less self-care time? Or maybe you lost your sense of self, your independence, the things that make you come alive.

For each thing you lost, name a few ways you can regain those things. Perhaps you can pursue projects you didn't have time for or commit to understanding yourself better. Maybe you lost your identity to the relationship and can start to explore who you are again.

Why can't Maeve move on?

It becomes clear that Maeve does not want to talk about anything other than Finn. It's as if talking about him keeps him alive and makes her alive by proxy. There's a kind of pleasure and excitement when talking about him, and I find myself getting drawn in. I eagerly await the sessions for more details about the forensic stalking of his social media. I find myself plotting conspiratorially with her as to what she should say next and how she should say it. One session, when she spends ten minutes reading me a text exchange from months ago, I have a sudden realisation. All this talking about Finn is stopping me from being able to do my work. It's like she's jumping up and down, pointing and saying, 'Look over here!' And it works – I'm looking – until I stop myself to think about what she's distracting me from.

This is a warning sign to me that all of this obsessing is probably her way of avoiding something. So I try to move the conversation away from Finn, to get a fuller sense of Maeve and who she is. Yet each time I inquire about work or family or friends, we end up back on Finn within a couple of minutes. It's exhausting, but clearly talking about him is doing something for Maeve; it's fulfilling a kind of purpose.

I realise that actually us talking about him and the reasons for the break-up is keeping her from moving on. Like an addict who cannot stop. Even though she knows it's over, it doesn't feel like she's fully accepted this. And when we're in a state of denial, we're usually avoiding the pain that comes with acceptance.

'It sounds,' I say to Maeve, 'with all the scenarios and texts you're curating, that you think you'll be able to win him back.' She nods sheepishly. 'But,' I continue, 'it doesn't sound like Finn wants to be won back. It sounds like there's nothing you can do.'

I'm being direct and maybe a little too challenging, but it feels as though Maeve is still clinging on to a fantasy of control and hasn't quite accepted her reality. Maeve has little control over this situation, yet her obsession and scheming is giving her a false sense that she can do something about it.

I say this to Maeve. Her cheeks start to flush and her eyes tear up.

'What would happen if you accepted that he was gone?' I ask.

'I can't,' she says, blinking away the tears. 'It would hurt too much.'

She coughs down her sadness and starts talking about the details of the last conversation they had and what she wished she'd said differently – straight back out of the feeling and into plotting mode. I deflate.

Because Maeve is so resistant to allowing in her grief, I start to wonder if this is about more than just Finn. There may be something else in her past that has been triggered by the break-up, which Maeve is finding hard to face.

What else is going on?

The way we respond to a break-up is influenced by how we're affected by rejection and failure. Break-ups can trigger core wounds of abandonment, rejection and loss. This means they can trigger a whole host of feelings we're not even aware of.

It's usually harder to process if there are particularly deep attachment wounds that have been opened by the break-up. You may be reliving a childhood experience of feeling rejected and struggle to get over your ex because you needed them to prove you were lovable.

Remember the 'moral defence' I mentioned earlier (see page 125)? That is the survival technique we use as children to remain close to our parents by believing that they are good and we are bad (because we need them to be good for our survival). It leads us to blame everything on ourselves and to need others to prove we're lovable.

When relationships end, our feelings of being bad or unlovable can get triggered all over again. We needed our partner's love to prove we're good, so without them we feel ugly, too much, ashamed, small, bad. Maybe them leaving us triggers a core belief we have about ourselves – that if only we'd been better, sexier, less needy, more attentive, maybe they would have stayed. Like dominoes, this might trigger memories of when our family made us feel rejected, when they were upset or annoyed or critical and we couldn't understand what we'd done wrong, which makes us feel even more shame and rejection. So, to get away from all these horrible feelings, we pine for that person, obsessing and longing for them, because when they left they took with them the part that made us feel like we're enough. What we're really longing for is proof that we are loved and good.

We're not really chasing them; we're chasing how they made us feel – worthy and good. The solution is to shift the moral defence, to learn that we are good, that our parents' flaws were not our fault, so we can feel whole on our own and not need others to confirm our worth.

You might not be aware of this, but that doesn't mean it isn't happening. If you can't get over someone, it's a clue that something deeper might have been stirred.

Maeve's breakthrough

Slowly, in the rare moments when we aren't talking about Finn, Maeve opens up more about her past. Her dad wasn't very interested in her when she was young. He did all the right things – playing games, buying presents, being around – but there was a disconnect. He always seemed to prefer her younger sister, who was funny and boyish and interested in football, just like he was. Maeve tried everything she could to make him like her; she'd pretend she was into sports, ask questions about his job, but he was always distracted, one eye on the TV as if she wasn't important enough to focus on. Then her sister would walk through the door and his face would light up. He'd switch off the television, grab a ball and off they'd trot together, leaving Maeve alone in the hallway, wondering why she wasn't being picked.

The only logical conclusion her child self could draw was that her sister must have been better than her. Not developed enough to understand that her dad's apathy was more about him than her, Maeve grew up believing that she was inferior, unlovable.

Then Finn came along and showered her with the adoration she'd been craving her whole life. His love came in the little moments. He'd make her morning coffee in her favourite mug, he'd rub cream into the spots on her back she couldn't reach, he'd watch *EastEnders* with her, even though it bored him. For Christmas one year, he hand-wrapped an advent calendar present for her for each of the twenty-five days, which she opened proudly in front of her jealous roommates. She knew where her place was with Finn; it was the first time she felt she really belonged.

As they got to know each other more, Maeve confessed to Finn about her competition with her sister, how she was convinced she was uglier and less interesting, and sometimes, in the dark pits of her mind, she wondered if Finn would swap if he had the chance. Finn laughed, not out of cruelty, but out of love. 'You'll always be my favourite,' he said. She savoured his words like they were nectar. For the first time she started to believe she was worthy of being cared about.

Then when Finn stopped helping around the house and left her to do everything on her own, it felt like she was losing her dad's attention all over again. She sought out the affair in an unconscious attempt to feel loved and important again.

When Finn left, all those feelings of standing alone in the hallway came rushing back. Except Maeve does not want to believe that she is inferior and unworthy, and accepting Finn's rejection would do that. So she stays in denial because, in an odd way, it's less painful than the alternative. By winning Finn back, she can regain control of his rejection – and her dad's – and prove that she is indeed worthy of love.

– *EXERCISE* –

If you feel stuck like Maeve and unable to move on from a break-up, something deeper might have been triggered.

First, think of any rejection or abandonment you faced in childhood. When's the earliest you felt this way? This could be a literal abandonment, like a parent leaving or dying, or an emotional abandonment. This could also be from siblings, teachers, school peers – anyone you were close to who made you feel rejected in some way.

Might the break-up have triggered any of these feelings or beliefs about yourself? With Maeve, the divorce may have triggered fears that people don't love her, that she is inferior and unlovable. This doesn't mean, however, that these beliefs and fears are true – something feeling true is not the same as it being true.

How do you accept and move on?

Maeve and I talk about what it felt like as that little girl, watching her dad choose her sister over her. She remembers the coldness, the anger, the longing for the warmth he was clearly capable of.

'The funny thing is,' Maeve says, 'I tried everything. I tried to be so many versions of myself, but still my dad wasn't interested.'

'A bit like you're trying to do with Finn,' I say.

Maeve laughs.

'Maybe it wasn't about me, the way my dad was. Maybe it wasn't anything I was doing. It's no way to treat your daughter – I'd never make mine feel like that,' she says, in touch with the unfairness of it all for the first time.

I have the urge to hug her, but I don't. It's a painful experience to connect to that vulnerability, but I also know that this is where healing can lie.

As we progress, Finn fades away from the forefront of her mind and the focus of the therapy. One session she comes in and starts talking about work instead of him. I'm surprised, and I go with it. Inevitably he comes back in, but I note the slight shift away from him. A few weeks later she's having a crisis of envy with her sister getting a new job and she doesn't mention Finn at all. Silently I register that the obsession is lessening.

As Maeve is becoming more aware of the deeper feelings the break-up triggered, the need to talk about Finn lessens. As she starts to realise that her dad's behaviour wasn't really about her, she starts to loosen the belief that there was something wrong with her, and doesn't yearn so much for Finn to prove she's lovable.

Accepting our parents' flaws is one of the most painful parts of therapy, but it's so vitally important that we do, because with that we can really grasp that there is nothing wrong with us. We were not bad or selfish or too much or not enough. We were perfectly OK; we were just raised by people and a society that were probably a little damaged themselves.

By empathising with the innocent little child we were, and still carry with us, we're accepting that our parents will never love us in the way we hoped. This brings a whole new level of grief. Grief for our child self who didn't get what they needed, and never will. It's a bitter truth that many of us spend our whole lives running away from, but accepting it can also free us.

Key steps to getting over someone

1. **Give yourself space to grieve.** There is no right way to do this, and it will take as long as it takes, but it's hard to truly move on and let go until you feel the pain of the loss. Give yourself permission to really feel it, however that might look for you.

2. **Refocus your energy on yourself.** Think about the parts of yourself you've lost to the relationship and try to rebuild them. Find your self-worth outside of that person by pursuing the things you care about and committing to yourself.

3. **Prioritise your pleasure and self-care.** You need to prove to yourself that you can be happy without them. Put your pleasure at the centre of your focus to show yourself that you'll be OK without them. This is

about finding a way to feel whole on your own. It's also important to treat yourself with compassion, which might be eating well, exercising, sleeping well. Care for yourself in the way you'd care for someone you love.

4. **Stop talking to your ex or about your ex.** Think of it like a fire you're trying to let burn out. The more you talk about them and talk to them, the more you're feeding the fire that's burning inside you and stopping you from moving on. It might be cold for a while, but over time you'll be able to build a new fire for yourself that is all yours.

5. **Rely on your friends and loved ones.** When we're feeling lonely after a break-up, filling the gap with friends can be a huge help, as it shows us we can have connection outside of the relationship. It's OK to rely on people – let yourself ask for help.

6. **Connect to the original wound.** Any feelings of rejection, powerlessness, grief or loneliness may also trigger a deeper wound. Try to get to the source of those feelings and connect to grief your inner child needs to feel.

CONCLUSION

You Don't Have to Suffer

I want to make it clear that, despite what you may think, and what I may have portrayed in this book, healing is not about suffering. Yes, sometimes you need to go through the pain in order to process it and stop it from negatively affecting your life, but healing is about letting go of suffering, which, as you'll see, some of us are reluctant to do.

Suffering can be addictive. Just as the brain can get addicted to substances, it can also get addicted to negative states and feelings. Stress and negative feelings release adrenaline and cortisol, which create a vicious cycle where we continue to chase the rush of those chemicals, so seek out more stress and suffering.

This is our body's attempt to keep the status quo. If you came from a home where you suffered, your brain might keep you in situations that cause suffering because it feels familiar. Your unconscious wants to maintain homeostasis – for things to stay the same – so if you've known suffering or chaos, chances are you'll seek it out because it feels familiar. We can get addicted to suffering in this way, even though it doesn't feel good. In a weird way, it feels safe and that's comforting. If pain tends to be your go-to solution – through self-harm, drinking until you feel sick, eating until you feel sick, being self-destructive, overworking, being constantly stressed, talking negatively to yourself, getting yourself into situations that keep you stuck and miserable – you might want to shift your focus to allow a little more pleasure into your life.

I've noticed this in my patients too. They come to me with highly stressful situations, like being in a toxic relationship or seeking out dangerous situations, but there's an excitement, a kind of charge to the pain they're in. I see it in people who are obsessive thinkers, driving themselves crazy by overthinking about a person or a situation and kind of enjoying the loop of anxiety (even though they recognise that it's ruining their lives). Some people are self-hating and depressed, but again there's a masochistic pleasure in beating themselves up in this way, as if there's a part of them that finds it oddly satisfying to self-flagellate. It's this pleasure that can make letting go of the suffering difficult.

To release the suffering you have to feel it, not hold onto it. It might feel like letting go is giving up control, but the need for control is the problem, not the solution.

I once went to my own therapist in the grips of stress and anxiety about a situation that was beyond my control. I had a difficult interaction with a friend who was pulling me into a drama and positioning me in a way that was making me angry and defensive. 'It's so unfair,' I lamented to my therapist, having read her the frustrated text I'd spent all night crafting. My therapist looked at me with the squinty eyes she saves for when she's about to say something that cuts through my bullshit and said, 'You're enjoying this, aren't you?' I stopped for a moment, alarmed because I knew she was right. I was suffering, but I was oddly excited and drawn in by it. 'What would happen if you let it go?' she asked. I thought about it and felt my shoulders come down from my ears. I sighed. 'That feels good, relaxing, like I can step out of the drama.' I decided not to reply to my friend, to disengage from the adrenaline-fuelled exchange I was caught up in, and to choose peace.

How to choose peace

First, you have to recognise the role you're playing in your own suffering. When you're stuck in anxious and depressive ways of thinking, it can feel like that negativity is caused by external things – our partners, our family, our job, the state of the world, etc. Of course, these things have a big effect on us, but we usually can't control those things. What we can change is our relationship to those things, by starting to acknowledge what we can control. The more you blame others and your circumstances, the less empowered you feel to change things. Yes, my friend was being totally unreasonable and infuriating, but I was choosing to engage with them. There is always a choice, even when you feel totally powerless. By walking away from the situation, I was reclaiming my power. Recognising the role you're playing in your own suffering can often be quite empowering, because if you are choosing suffering, you can also choose to suffer less.

Now, I don't mean we should all 'just be happy'; obviously it isn't that easy. I'm also not trying to victim blame – being in an abusive situation is not your fault, and neither were any of the things that happened to you as a child.

That said, I think victim terminology can be disempowering because it makes it seem as though there's nothing we can do. Getting out of abusive situations is incredibly challenging and scary and requires great strength and support, but it is possible for many. This isn't about blame, but about locating our power even when we feel totally powerless. By recognising the choices we are making, we can find our own solutions.

Choose peace. When you're suffering, you might feel that you have no power at all, especially if you're feeling depressed and lonely. But your thoughts are not necessarily true. There may be things you can do; you might just not want to do them.

So if you're stuck and feeling powerless, ask yourself: how would I choose peace?

Why therapy works (if you let it)

You've (hopefully) learnt by now that relationships are essential to us humans. They are essential to our suffering, and also to our healing.

Healing on your own can feel lonely sometimes. You're going through your past, having new and uncomfortable feelings, trying to show up differently in your life, and you're still expected to go on with things as normal. Behind your smile people can't see what you're going through. But it doesn't have to be this way. Healing can, and should, take place through relationships.

We are also wounded through relationships. Think about most of the things that were difficult in childhood; they almost always involve relationship to another: death, abuse, absence, neglect, criticism, not having your emotional needs met, being too close, not being close enough. Relationships have the power to hurt us deeply, but they are also how we heal.

This is why therapy can be so transformational. You experience what it's like to be in a relationship where someone listens to you, tries to understand you, creates space for you, challenges you with compassion and unconditionally supports you. Many of you may never have had a relationship like this. I know I hadn't.

Therapy can be a reparative experience. Those feelings you were told not to have are shown to someone, and they don't leave you or shout at you for it. They stay. This is a profound lesson. To have the experience of being brave enough to get angry or cry in front of someone and realise that they can bear your tears, and that they still come back week after week, is reparative beyond words. You're learning that you are OK as you are. You can be vulnerable and messy and 'wrong', and someone will still be there.

Therapy isn't the only relationship that can heal

Let me be very clear: this does NOT mean that you should become a therapist to your friends and lovers. To all you fixers who hear this and think, 'Great, she's giving me permission to try to heal everyone I'm in a relationship with,' this is not what I mean!

What I mean is that you heal *yourself* through relationships. Every time you show a feeling you would have previously been too afraid to share, set a boundary you've always struggled with, advocate for yourself, take a moment to reflect before reacting, show your more sensitive side to someone, and you get a positive response, you are healing. And you are doing this by being different with the people around you and learning that it's OK. You're rewiring your survival system by learning that it is safe to do or show the thing you were afraid of. And if you don't get a positive response, think carefully about the kind of relationship you want with that person.

Outside of therapy, this kind of healing relationship is still possible, though it will be less one-way. It can exist within a supportive friendship, a relationship where you're both learning to be different or a group, such as a sharing circle or a yoga class. Anywhere you can be vulnerable, where you can fully express yourself and be accepted, is a place of healing.

This does not have to be a solo process, and nor should it be. It's OK to ask for help. It's OK to need people. Let your most vulnerable self be loved. It deserves to be known.

Why is change so difficult?

Most people come to therapy because they want something to change. However, what I often find is that, while people want things to be different, they also want things to be exactly the same. You might say you want to change, and I'm sure you really believe you do, but somehow you're still stuck. This conundrum was summed up perfectly by a patient who once said to me, 'I want things to be different, but I don't want anything to change.'

I see this as a tug of war. There's a part of you that wants to change and a part of you that doesn't; each side is pulling hard, leaving you stuck in the middle, not really moving. We could try to pull harder on the end that wants to change, but the part that doesn't will probably get more scared and up the ante.

Rather than beating yourself up for this, try to get curious and think about why – why might there be a part of you that doesn't want to change? Why might you be sabotaging or resisting things? What might you be afraid to feel, admit or accept in yourself? What might you be gaining by staying in this position? To really change, you first have to meet that stuck place, and then try to unstick it.

All change involves loss, and most of us don't want to face loss, so we stay in relationships that aren't working to avoid breaking up, get stuck in jobs that aren't making us happy, keep up with friends we don't have anything in common with any more, and all because we don't want to let go. Or, on the flip side, some of us walk away before we've got to know someone, fall out with friends or cut people off for making small mistakes, and this is also usually motivated by a fear of loss – 'I'll leave you before you leave me.'

Many of us don't realise how resistant we are to change. But that unconscious resistance is tugging hard, keeping us in the same place we keep saying we don't want to be in. Remember, we are wired for safety, not for happiness. What we learnt during our most formative years is familiar and still feels safest to our unconscious selves, even though those very safety mechanisms are keeping us stuck.

How to change

First, you have to believe that change is possible, and for that, you have to recognise that you are contributing to your problems. That's not to say that other people aren't to blame – often it's other people who made us this way – but as adults it's up to us to take responsibility for our lives. Many people come into therapy feeling powerless, as if there's nothing they can do. They find fault with everyone else, thinking that if only their partner, bosses, friends, family, kids, dog were different, they could be happy. If this sounds like you, I'm sorry to break it to you, but not only are those people unlikely to change, they're also unlikely to solve all your problems. What might shift your problems is you.

That doesn't mean that other people aren't a major source of distress in our lives. People can be awful and cause us great pain. But we are not powerless in the face of that. We can change the way we show up in those relationships, set boundaries, walk away. By staying and doing nothing, we are choosing pain for ourselves.

It's a bitter pill to swallow, but it's also the pill that will free you.

Once you realise you have more choices than you thought, you can start to make things different for yourself. Taking responsibility for the pain you're causing yourself is difficult; it's something I wrestle with often myself. But when you make others responsible for your life, you lose the power to make changes, and this leaves you feeling like the powerless little child you once were.

Most people don't realise how much of their power they give away. Letting others influence them, seeking advice from everyone else, waiting for permission to do things, expecting others to change to meet their needs, blaming their lack of change on things outside of their control – all these things leave us feeling like passengers in our own life, and generally keeps us stuck. Taking responsibility for yourself is hard work, especially if you've been raised by dominating and overbearing parents. But once you realise you have the power to make decisions, to say no, to go for opportunities, to speak up for yourself, your life will become far more peaceful.

So I encourage you to make the change you're afraid of – set the boundaries, leave the relationships; whatever the thing is you're afraid to do but know deep down you should. That is likely the thing that will change your life the most.

Why it takes time

Many people come into therapy expecting instant results. I have to point out that change does not happen overnight. You've spent your whole life with entrenched patterns; they aren't going to shift after one session. They're disappointed. They want a quick fix, a magic pill, for me to wave my wand and take away all their problems.

I know you probably don't want to hear this, but change takes time, because repetition is essential for any change we want to make. We want the new behaviour to become the stronger neural pathway – the route our brain takes without thinking. But we're changing years and years of well-trodden paths here, so we have to do it over and over and over again.

If, when you were younger, you tried being vulnerable and this made you feel rejected, your brain would have created a neural pathway that made you shut down or change the conversation every time someone asked you something that made you feel vulnerable. Remember, rejection can feel like a threat to survival, so our survival instincts close down the vulnerability path and choose the path of avoidance instead.

That neural pathway (vulnerability = avoidance) will be very strong by now, like a well-defined ski slope that's been skied down a million times. It's the safer route, the one you've learnt will keep you alive. Your brain is interested in saving time and resources, so this path becomes automatic and deeply entrenched.

Now, your partner or a therapist asks you to be more open with them. That's a bit like going completely off-piste down fresh virgin snow. Not only does it not feel safe, it's also completely unfamiliar. So, let's say you're feeling brave and you force yourself to open up a bit and share some deeper feelings. Even if it goes well and doesn't feel as scary as you'd thought, your brain will still automatically go back to the well-trodden slope next time. So the next time, even though you've successfully made a change, your brain will return to the more familiar ski slope and avoid the difficult conversation.

That's why repetition is essential for any change we want to make. We want to repeat the new behaviour so many times that it becomes the stronger neural pathway – the easiest, automatic path.

The good news is that our adult brains are still changeable. While our brain stops developing around the age of twenty-one, neuroscience shows that brain plasticity remains into old age (even though it becomes harder to change the older we are), and therefore change is very possible. So if you repeat it enough, the new path will become second nature, and in time you'll find yourself easily opening up without even having to think about it.

Another reason why we might need to go over things a few times is because we're trying to help our mind feel safe enough to face what feels scary. Let's be realistic, if you've spent years and years believing it's not safe to admit you're jealous or show anger or be vulnerable, you're not going to suddenly be able to express those things. It takes time to feel safe.

My job as a therapist is to help people feel as safe as possible, which means taking our time. As someone who likes to go quickly and is always rushing, I find this a struggle – as a therapist and in my own therapy. People want to get better as quickly as possible, and I want to help them do that. But we can't rush safety. Some people feel safe immediately and can jump in. Others take years before they can go deep. It takes as long as it takes.

I was reminded of this with Alva, the *Candy Crush* addict. She was frustrated at herself because she could feel she was avoiding something, and I was finding this frustrating too. 'Just let yourself feel it,' I wanted to say to her. Yet every time we'd come close to the feeling, her eyes would fill, then she'd change the subject and move us away from the sadness.

This dance went on for months, and when I pointed it out she sighed, exasperated.

'I can feel I'm avoiding the pain. It's annoying – I know if I just let myself feel it then I wouldn't be so stuck. This process is annoyingly slow.'

'It sounds like you're in a rush,' I said.

'Yeah, I want to feel better. I don't want to be stuck any more.'

Alva's hands were in fists, as if she wanted to bash through to the pain but the pain wasn't playing ball. It was still in hiding, because it wasn't safe yet.

To get a better idea of what was going on inside her, I asked Alva to describe what she was feeling in her body.

She explained that there was a ball in her chest that was covered in chains, impenetrable. The ball, she described, was fragile, like an egg.

'Well, we have a choice then,' I said. 'We can try to rush things, to hammer down the chains and break open the egg.'

She shook her head. 'That doesn't sound nice.'

'No. Or we can give the egg what it needs.'

'What does it need?' she asked me, eyes wide like a child.

'You tell me.'

'Something gentle, I think.' Her fists unclenched. 'Something softer, less scary, so it knows it's safe.'

When she left after that session I let myself cry. Alva had reminded me of my own vulnerability, how force can do more harm than good. I, too, had been forcing myself to heal quickly, frustrated at my own defensiveness. Alva had reminded me that I also needed something slow and tender. I've always thought of my version of a fragile egg as a tiny child inside me locked behind a door. I've tried, many times, to bash down the door and every time she's run and hidden away. What has worked is slowly, inch by inch, opening the door until she feels safe enough to come out.

We shouldn't bash through the chains or force down the doors – they are the things that are keeping us safe. If we do that, the egg will crack rather than hatch. What we need is to go slowly, to let the feelings come up only when we feel safe enough to handle them.

You'll never be finished, and that's OK

Healing is never really done. You never fully understand yourself or battle all your demons. You're never finished, and that is part of the beauty of it. Different lessons will come to you at different times in your life – some problems presented in this book might be relevant to you now, others might be relevant in ten years. As long as you stay curious and open to understanding yourself, you're on the right track.

You might have read all this and imagined that I have it all figured out. It's taken me a long time to learn the lessons in this book, and even then, after years of therapy and studying to be a psychotherapist, I still struggle with a lot of it. We are all human and therefore necessarily imperfect and vulnerable. Even the person you think has it all sussed will have their insecurities.

Healing is not something you complete. Many years into therapy, I'm still having a-ha moments, pushing away difficult feelings, denying my vulnerability, struggling to speak up, messing up in relationships. Knowing all of this is not a short cut for going through the process of healing; in fact, sometimes it makes it more complicated because you think you understand something intellectually, but emotionally you're not there yet.

All the theory in the world is not the same as going through the process. You have to grieve for what you never had, get stuck in the in-between phase of knowing you need to change but not wanting to, feel the prickly terror of having a difficult conversation for the first time, and let yourself get mad and sad and everything in between. You have to learn to accept people, and yourself, and – the hardest part of all – really learn to love yourself along the way.

Reading about it is useful, but it isn't the same as doing it. In a way, this book is the tip of the iceberg. Now you just need to take what you've learnt, be brave and dive underneath the surface.

book and seeing them [illegible]

[illegible]

[illegible] many years into [illegible]

[illegible] in the process [illegible]

[illegible] and everything in between. [illegible]

[illegible]

RESOURCES

If you're feeling distressed right now and want to talk to someone, you can contact 24-hour helplines with people trained to listen to you.

Samaritans. To talk about anything that is upsetting you, you can contact Samaritans 24 hours a day, 365 days a year. You can call 116 123 (free), email jo@samaritans.org or visit some branches in person. You can also call the Samaritans Welsh Language Line on 0808 164 0123 (7 p.m.–11 p.m. every day).

National Suicide Prevention Helpline UK offers a supportive listening service to anyone with thoughts of suicide. Call 0800 689 5652 (6 p.m.–3.30 a.m. every day).

Shout. If you would prefer not to talk but want some mental health support, you could text SHOUT to 85258. Shout offers a confidential 24/7 text service providing support if you are in crisis and need immediate help.

ENDNOTES

1 Felitti, V. J., Anda, R. F., Nordenberg, D., Williamson, D. F., Spitz, A. M., Edwards, V., Koss, M. P. and Marks, J. S. (1998). 'Relationship of childhood abuse and household dysfunction to many of the leading causes of death in adults. The Adverse Childhood Experiences (ACE) Study', *American Journal of Preventive Medicine*, 14(4), 245-258.

2 Van der Kolk, B. A. (2014). *The Body Keeps the Score: Brain, Mind, and Body in the Healing of Trauma* (New York: Viking).

3 Fairbairn, W. R. D. (1944). 'Endopsychic structure considered in terms of object-relationships', *The International Journal of Psychoanalysis* 25, 70–93.

4 Fincham, G. W., Strauss, C., Montero-Marin, J., and Cavanagh, K. (2023). 'Effect of breathwork on stress and mental health: A meta-analysis of randomised-controlled trials', *Scientific Reports* 13(1), 432.

5 Kuzminskaite, E., Penninx, B. W. J. H., van Harmelen, A. L., Elzinga, B. M., Hovens, J. G. F. M., and Vinkers, C. H. (2021). 'Childhood Trauma in Adult Depressive and Anxiety Disorders: An Integrated Review on Psychological and Biological Mechanisms in the NESDA Cohort', *Journal of Affective Disorders* 283, 179-191.

6 Winnicott, D. W. (1991). *Playing and Reality* (London: Psychology Press).

7 Van der Kolk, B. A. (1996). 'The body keeps score: Approaches to the psychobiology of posttraumatic stress disorder'. In van der Kolk, B.A., McFarlane, A. C. and Weisaeth, L. (eds.), *Traumatic Stress: The Effects of Overwhelming Experience on Mind, Body, and Society*, 214–241. (New York: The Guilford Press).

8 Levine, P. A. (1997). *Waking the Tiger: Healing Trauma* (Berkeley, California: North Atlantic Books).

9 Kendall-Tackett, K. (2009). 'Psychological Trauma and Physical Health: A Psychoneuroimmunology Approach to Etiology of Negative Health Effects and Possible Interventions', *Psychological Trauma: Theory, Research, Practice, and Policy*, 1(1), 35. Also Resick, P. A. (2014). *Stress and Trauma* (London: Psychology Press).

10 Baker, H. S. and Baker, M. N. (1987). 'Heinz Kohut's self psychology: an overview', *The American Journal of Psychiatry*, 144 (1), 1–9.

11 Fairbairn, W. R. D. (1943). 'The repression and the return of bad objects (with special reference to the "war neuroses")', *British Journal of Medical Psychology*, 19, 327–41.

12 Winnicott, D. W. (1960). 'Ego distortion in terms of true and false self' in *The Maturational Process and the Facilitating Environment: Studies in the Theory of Emotional Development* (New York: International Universities Press, Inc), 140–57.

13 Flückiger, C., Del Re, A. C., Wampold, B. E., and Horvath, A. O. (2018). 'The alliance in adult psychotherapy: A meta-analytic synthesis', *Psychotherapy*, 55(4), 316–340.

14 Fisher, H. E., Brown, L. L., Aron, A., Strong, G. and Mashek,

D. (2010). 'Reward, addiction, and emotion regulation systems associated with rejection in love', *Journal of Neurophysiology*, 104(1), 51-60.

15 Freud, S. (1920) *Beyond the Pleasure Principle. The Standard Edition of the Complete Psychological Works of Sigmund Freud*, 18, 1-64.

16 Holmes, J. (2014). *John Bowlby and Attachment Theory* (London: Routledge).

17 Perel, E. (2006). *Mating in Captivity: Reconciling the Erotic and the Domestic* (New York: HarperCollins), p. 272.

18 Berne, E. (1961). *Transactional analysis in psychotherapy: A systematic individual and social psychiatry* (Souvenir Press).

19 Kübler-Ross, E. and Kessler, D. (2005). *On Grief and Grieving: Finding the Meaning of Grief Through the Five Stages of Loss* (New York: Simon & Schuster).

ACKNOWLEDGEMENTS

To my patients, past and present, I continue to learn every day from your courage and vulnerability. I know how scary it is to sit on the other side of the couch, it is my true privilege to sit alongside you.

To anyone who follows or engages with *Your Pocket Therapist*, never in my wildest dreams did I think I would connect with and help so many people, I'm so grateful for the community we've built. It's inspiring to see just how willing people are to engage with themselves and their relationships on a deep level – it's nice to know I'm not the only one obsessed with therapy and psychology! I will endeavour to carry on trying to help you learn about yourself and your relationships until you're sick of me.

To Matilda, speaking of therapy obsession, how lucky am I to have an agent who's as obsessed with therapy as I am? You've made me feel supported throughout every step of this process, and your directness and honesty has made the book and my writing infinitely better, I'm excited to see where your wisdom and ideas will take me in the future and, if nothing else, continue to chat therapy until we're bored (unlikely). I'd also like to thank the rest of the WME team – Florence Dodd, Sabrina Taitz, Adela McBride.

To my UK editor, Jess Duffy, you were the first person to envisage this book and see the potential in YPT. Collaborating with you has been a dream, I felt immediately understood by you, and consistently supported throughout the entire process. Thanks for believing in me, giving me ideas and expertise while also giving me the freedom to write the book I wanted. And to the brilliant team at Orion Spring – Carina Bryan, Helena Fouracre, Ellen Turner, Paul Stark, Katie Horrocks, Frances Rooney, Helen Ewing, Jessica Hart, Jennifer Wilson, Pippa Wright and Anna Valentine – and to Lauren Bahorun for your help producing the audiobook – there are so many more people involved in writing a book than you realise, it truly takes a village and I'm honoured that this book has been raised by a group of such talented and hardworking people. Huge thanks also go to my US editor, Anna Montague, for your enthusiastic and gentle manner, and the whole team at Dey Street.

To my colleagues, tutors and supervisors at the Guild of Psychotherapy, thank you for the support, intellectual stimulation, and freedom to develop my own practice and identity as a therapist. This book is a combined result of all the teachings that I have learnt from each of you (though apologies if I've butchered most of them).

To readers of my early, and questionable, writing: Mum for teaching me the rules, James Wheale for teaching me that there are no rules (and giving me the courage to do any of this in the first place), to Chris Hemmings, for being my most honest and direct friend (and my biggest champion), to my dearest friends and colleagues Caitlin O'Donnell and Dawn Finzi for the years of psychological debates, taking the time to think with me about what I wanted to say, and how, and letting me benefit off the wisdom of your experience on my (very rainy) California writing retreat, and Chris Fish for helping me come up with the characters and helping me during the writing process.

To my Book Klub, for being the first round of readers even though most of you had to read it on your phones, your insights were invaluable. Special thanks to Pete for being thoughtful enough to get it professionally printed and bound – you're the best.

I'm lucky enough to have wonderful friends in my life, who give me both depth and silliness in equal measure, Emma Marchant, Rakhee Patel, Zoe Zietman, Emma Wyeth, Kira Pillai, Ellie Milone, Olly Needham, James Wheale, Chris Hemmings, Becca Beckley, Tom Deering, Brismas crew (for spending the best part of a year helping me think of subtitles), all the Whimsy lot and many more – I love you all.

To Nicola, you've taught me more about therapy than I could have learnt in any book or training. The only reason I'm so passionate about therapy is because I have experienced firsthand the way that it can change your life, and that is largely thanks to you, and my therapists that came before, Els and Paul. You've shown me how to contain, challenge, provoke, love (and hate), and all while maintaining tenderness and reverie. Not to be too hyperbolic, but this book would not exist without you, and my life would be significantly worse.

To my wonderful extended family, ZimRoSis, thank you for all your enthusiasm, support, constant analysis of family dynamics and nonstop crosswords.

To Mum for all the inspiring and eye-opening therapy chats, I've learnt so much from your wisdom and passion, and to Dad for keeping us from drowning under all the 'psychobabble'. Mum – thanks for reading every essay I've ever written and being the biggest champion of my writing.

Dad – thanks for being my best pal, being so keen to read the book and giving your 'man from the Clapham omnibus' insights. To both of you for being frighteningly intelligent and fostering a thirst for reading and writing (even though I have failed to inherit your crossword skills), for making me believe I can achieve anything and holding me when things don't go according to plan.

To my sister, Katie, getting to be loved by you is the greatest thing that has ever happened to me, knowing that you're in my corner has made me a more open, loving and confident person. You've taught me how to be vulnerable and soft and silly. Thank you for holding me, for seeing me, for making me laugh, for spending a lifetime analysing all our family dynamics, and never failing to be by my side. I couldn't love you more, even when I hate you, and I'm eternally grateful I get to have you as my sister and best friend.

To Pete, for surprising me in all the best ways and showing me the kind of love I've always dreamed of but didn't know existed. This is it now.

Lastly Albie, my co-star and in-house furry therapist. I'm glad the world gets to experience your gentle and grounding nature that I benefit from on a daily basis. The unconditional love of a dog is possibly the most therapeutic thing a person can experience, if you can't afford a therapist, get a dog instead.

ABOUT THE AUTHOR

Annie Zimmerman, PhD, is a psychotherapist, writer and academic. Annie began posting her life-changing insights from the therapy room on TikTok and Instagram as @your_pocket_therapist in 2021 and has since amassed a large and dedicated following who return to her content for advice on everything from attachment styles and inner child work to making peace with your body.